中醫五臟病機了

Pathomechanisms of the Five Viscera

Zhōng Yī Wǔ Zàng Bìng Jī Xué

心病之病機

Pathomechanisms of the

HEART

Xīn Bìng Zhī Bìng Jī

Yán Shí-Lín, Lǐ Zhèng-Huá

严石林, 李正华

With the Assistance of

Yán Yǎn 严俨, Lǐ Wěi Hóng 李炜弘, Zhāng Chí 张驰, Gāo Fēng 高峰

Edited by Eric Brand and Zhāng Yǔhuán 张宇环
Translated by Sabine Wilms and Wáng Yīng 王英

Paradigm Publications

Taos, New Mexico 2005

Pathomechanisms of the Five Viscera
Volume 1
Pathomechanisms of the Heart

Yán Shí Lín 严石林　　Lǐ Zhèng-Huá 李正华

Translated by Wáng Yīng 王英 and Sabine Wilms
Edited by Eric Brand and Zhāng Yǔ Huán

Copyright © 2005 Paradigm Publications
202 Bendix Drive, Taos, NM 87571
www.paradigm-pubs.com
Distributed by Redwing Book Company
www.redwingbooks.com

Library of Congress Cataloging-in-Publication Data

Yan, Shi Lin, 1943-
   [Zhong Yi Wu Zang Bing Ji Xue: Xin Bing Zhi Bing Ji. English]
   Pathomechanisms of the five viscera: pathomechanisms of the heart / Yan
   Shi Lin, Li Zheng-Hua ; with
   the assistance of Yan Yan ... [et al.] ; translated by Wang Ying and
   Sabine Wilms ; edited by Eric Brand and Zhang Yu Huan.
     p. ; cm.
   Includes bibliographical references and index.
   ISBN 0-912111-79-8
   1. Heart--Pathophysiology. 2. Medicine, Chinese.   I. Li,
Zheng-Hua,
   1942-   . II. Brand, Eric, 1978-   . III. Wiseman, Nigel. IV.
Title.
   [DNLM: 1. Heart--physiopathology. 2. Medicine, Chinese
Traditional.
   WG 200 Y21z 2005a]
   RC682.9.Y36125 2005
   616.1'2--dc22

2005023189

Library of Congress Number: 2005023189

International Standard Book Number (ISBN): 0-912111-79-8

Printed in the United States of America

Table of Contents

Council of Oriental Medical Publishers

Designation

This work is a whole-text translation of the Chinese text, *Zhī Xīn Bìng Bìng Jī* 心 病 病 机 by Yán Shí Lín 严石林. English terminology conforms to Wiseman and Feng, *Practical Dictionary of Chinese Medicine* published by Paradigm Publications.

Pathomechanisms of the Heart

心病病机

The heart holds the office of monarch and governs the blood and vessels of the entire body. It transports the nutrients and irrigates the four limbs and the hundred bones. Internally, it moistens the five viscera and six bowels; externally, it nourishes the skin, hair, and interstices. The heart also governs the spirit-mind. Thus, it regulates a person's essence-spirit, thought, and consciousness. The heart is the great governor of the five viscera and the six bowels; thus, it supervises the functions of the bowels and viscera and commands the entire body.

The heart corresponds to the vessels, its bloom is in the face, it opens at the tongue, and it stands in exterior-interior relationship with the small intestine. Irregularities in the physiological functioning of the heart manifest mainly in two types of pathomechanisms: abnormalities of the blood and vessels and changes in the spirit-mind.

心者君主之官，主一身之血脉，输送营养物质，灌溉四肢百骸，内润五脏六腑，外养皮毛腠理；又主神志，调节人的精神、思维、意识活动，统摄脏腑功能，主宰全身，为五脏六腑之大主。心在体为脉，其华在面，开窍于舌，与小肠互为表里。心的生理功能失调，常表现为血脉异常和神志改变两类病机变化。

1. Abnormalities of the Blood and Vessels

When the functions of the heart become irregular, severe pathologies may develop. When its ability to transport blood and to govern the vessels is impaired, the blood is deprived of nourishment in the heart viscus itself, as well as in the head and face, the four limbs, and all the organs. This produces a series of pathomechanisms.

Heart Viscus: When the heart viscus is deprived of nourishment, the governing pathology involves stirring in the heart. In this category, the failure of the blood to nourish the heart and the inhibited movement of blood can manifest in symptoms such as heart palpitations and fearful throbbing, and emptiness in the heart or heart pain. An abnormally fast or slow heartbeat may cause changes in the frequency, rhythm, or strength of the pulse. This can manifest in a pulse that is rapid, slow, vacuous, replete, slippery, rough, skipping (rapid and irregularly interrupted), bound, or intermittent (regularly interrupted).

Head and face: The blood vessels become full when blood and qì surge upwards. This results in redness in the face and eyes or red lips, as well as in redness, pain, and sores or ulcers on the tip of the tongue. Frenetic movement of blood may lead to blood ejection and spontaneous external bleeding. If blood and qì are deprived of nourishment and the blood vessels lose fullness, the result is a pale white or withered-yellow complexion with pale white lips and tongue. If the movement of blood is inhibited, blood stasis in the vessels presents externally with the color of the static blood; this manifests in a somber or soot-black complexion, green-blue or purple lips and tongue, or in stasis macules or stasis speckles on the tongue.

Four limbs: If the blood in the vessels is exuberant and heat is sufficient, there will be vexing heat in the four limbs and heat in the palms and soles. If the blood in the vessels is congealed by cold, the reduction of heat may lead to counterflow cold of the limbs, cold pain in the hands and feet, and purple or dark nails.

Entire Body: In cases where all the bowels and viscera of the body suffer from a lack of supply of blood and qì and are deprived of nourishment, many manifestations of lowered and weakened organ functions can be observed.

血脉异常

心的功能失调，很大一类病变为不能输布血液，主持血脉的功能异常，引起心脏自身、头面、四肢及全身脏腑血液失养而出现一系列病机变化。

心脏自身失养，病变以心动不安为主：其中血不养心，血行不畅，可见心悸怔忡，或心中空虚，心痛等症；心跳过速或过缓，引起脉搏的跳动频率、节律、强度等发生变化，可见数、迟、虚、实、滑、涩、促、结、代等脉象改变。

头面部位，当血气上冲时，血脉充盈，则为面红目赤，唇红，舌尖红赤、疼痛、溃烂；迫血妄行则为吐血、衄血；当血气失养时，血脉失充，又为面色淡白，萎黄，唇舌淡白；当血行不畅时，血脉瘀滞，瘀血之色外现，又见面色晦暗、黧黑，唇舌青紫，或舌有瘀斑瘀点。

四肢部分，血脉充盛时，热能充足，则四肢烦热，手足心发烧；血脉寒凝时，热能减少，则四肢逆冷，手足冷痛，爪甲紫暗。

全身脏腑失却血气供养，可见脏腑功能低下、衰退的各种表现。

Summary of Abnormalities of the Blood and Vessels

1. Heart Viscus
   Heart palpitations: Heart palpitations, fearful throbbing, emptiness in the heart, shortness of breath, and heart pain
   Abnormally fast or slow heartbeat: A pulse that is rapid, slow, vacuous, replete, slippery, rough, skipping, bound or intermittent
2. Head and Face
   Fullness in the blood vessels: Redness in the face and eyes, red painful lips and tongue, possibly with blood ejection or spontaneous external bleeding
   Loss of fullness in the blood vessels: Pale white or withered-yellow complexion, pale white lips and tongue
   Static blood in the vessels: Somber or soot black complexion, blue-green or purple lips and tongue, possibly with stasis macules or stasis speckles
3. Four Limbs
   Heat vexation or counterflow cold
4. Entire Body
   Lowered or weakened functions of the bowels and viscera

血脉失常

心脏
　　心悸不安 —— 心悸怔忡，心中空虚，气短心痛。
　　过速过缓 —— 数、迟、虚、实、滑、涩、促、结、代。
头面
　　血脉充盈 —— 面红目赤，唇舌红赤疼痛，或吐血衄血。
　　血脉失充 ——面色淡白，萎黄，唇舌淡白。
　　血脉凝滞 —— 面色晦暗、黧黑，唇舌青紫，或瘀斑瘀点。
四肢
　　烦热或逆冷。
全身
　　脏腑功能低下、衰退。

2.   Changes in the Spirit-Mind

In Chinese medicine, pathologies of the essence-spirit and affect-mind are ascribed to the heart. When the heart fails to govern the spirit-mind, the functions and activities of the essence-spirit, thoughts, and consciousness become irregular. This pathomechanism manifests as a heart spirit deprived of nourishment, a harassed heart spirit, or an ungoverned heart spirit.

If the heart spirit is deprived of nourishment, it is unable to govern and control the ordinary activities of the thoughts and consciousness; this often leads to a disquieted heart spirit. This may present with a disquieted state of mind, unfocused thinking, and mental listlessness or reduced memory capacity.

If the heart spirit is harassed by disease evils, there will be stirring of the heart. In mild cases, this will manifest as heart vexation, insomnia, and profuse dreaming. In severe cases, it will give rise to mental derangement or possibly to agitation. This presents with vexation and agitation, manic raving and cursing, and hitting people and breaking things regardless of who is present. It may also result in ceaseless joy and laughter. Alternatively, it may present with deep withdrawal and little speech, manifesting in an indifferent expression, deep silence and lack of communication, deranged speech, alternating spells of crying and laughing, and feeble-mindedness.

If the heart spirit has suffered severe damage, the spirit-mind will be ungoverned, causing the heart spirit to float astray. In mild cases, this manifests as somnolence, abstraction, and drowsiness. In severe cases, it manifests with an unclear spirit-mind, sudden collapse, delirious speech, and frenetic stirring.

神志改变

人的精神情志病变，中医归属于心。心不主神志，精神、思维、意识等功能活动失调，可见心神失养、心神受扰和心神无主等病机变化.

心神失养，不能主持正常的思维意识活动，常致心神不宁，可见心绪不安，思想不集中，精神萎靡，记忆力减退等症。

心神受到病邪干扰，心动不安，轻者表现为心烦，失眠，多梦；重者引起精神错乱，或为躁动不安，表现为烦躁不宁，狂言怒骂，打人毁物，不避亲疏，喜笑不休；或为沉静少言，表现为表情淡漠，沉默寡言，语言错乱，时哭时笑，呆痴。

心神严重受损，神志无主，心神浮越，轻者为嗜睡，恍惚，朦胧。重者为神志不清，突然倒仆，谵语，妄动。

Summary of Pathological Changes in the Spirit-Mind

1. Heart Spirit Deprived of Nourishment
   Disquieted heart spirit, manifesting in pathoconditions of mental disquiet, inability to concentrate, and reduced memory capacity.
2. Harassed Heart Spirit
   Mild cases: Heart vexation, insomnia, profuse dreaming.
   Severe cases: Mental derangement.
   > *Vexation and agitation*: Vexation and agitation, manic raving and cursing, hitting people and breaking things regardless of who is present
   > *Deep withdrawal*: Indifferent expression, deep silence and lack of communication, alternating crying and laughing, and feeblemindedness.
3. Heart Spirit Floating Astray
   Mild cases: Somnolence, abstraction, drowsiness.
   Severe cases: Unclear spirit-mind, sudden collapse, delirious speech and frenetic stirring.

神志病变

心神失养
　　心神不宁，可见心绪不安，思想不集中，记忆力减退等症。
心神受扰
　　轻者——心烦，失眠，多梦。
　　重者——精神错乱
　　烦躁——烦躁不宁，狂言怒骂，打人毁物，不避亲疏。
　　沉静——表情淡漠，沉默寡言，时哭时笑，呆痴。
心神浮越
　　轻者——嗜睡，恍惚，朦胧。
　　重者——神志不清，突然倒仆，谵语妄动。

Overview of Pathomechanisms of the Heart

Heart disorders are primarily caused by external contraction of the six excesses and by internal damage from the seven affects. Of the six excesses, wind, cold, dampness, and heat are most likely to invade the heart. Heart disorders are easily caused by internal damage from the seven affects, particularly from sorrow, joy, anxiety, and thought. In addition, the following factors can all lead to various pathological changes in the heart: constitutional insufficiency, excessive taxation fatigue, dietary irregularities, a predilection for fatty and sweet foods, an inhibited qì dynamic, phlegm turbidity causing internal obstruction, an internal collection of dampness, upward invasion of water qì, collection of static blood, chronic and severe illness, a lack of treatment or inappropriate treatment, and the transmission of disorders from the other organs.

The pathomechanisms of the heart are best categorized under the two major headings of vacuity and repletion, in order to distinguish between the conditions of exuberance or debility of right and evil qì.

The *Huáng Dì Nèi Jīng* ("Yellow Emperor's Inner Canon") contains a discussion of "heart vacuity," beginning with the statement that "thought and preoccupation damage the heart." This statement is found in the *Sù Wèn* ("Plain Questions") chapter, "Treatise on the Engenderment of the Five Viscera."

Huá Tuó's *Zhōng Zàng Jīng* ("Central Treasury Canon"), from the Hàn Dynasty, is the first text to include a separate chapter discussing the heart viscus in terms of vacuity and repletion, cold and heat, life and death, and smoothness and counterflow. Mentioning "heart qì exuberance," "heart qì repletion," "heart vacuity," and similar terms, it discusses the pathomechanisms of heart disorders from the angles of vacuity and repletion, exuberance and debility.

Wáng Shū-Hé's *Mài Jīng* ("Pulse Canon"), from the Jìn Dynasty, describes the pathomechanisms of "heart repletion" and "heart vacuity" in even greater clarity. The chapter, "Feeling the Pulses at Man's Prognosis (*rén yíng*) [ST-9], Spirit Gate (*shén mén*) [HT-7] and Qì Opening [Wrist Pulse] in Front and Back," states:

> "In cases of heart repletion, when the pulses at the inch opening on the left hand [in this text known as Man's Prognosis (*rén yíng*) [ST-9]] reflect yīn repletion, this is [a disease of] the hand reverting yīn channel. The patient will suffer from oppression, inhibited bowel movements, abdominal fullness, heaviness in the four limbs, generalized heat effusion, and stomach distention.

> In cases of heart vacuity, when the pulses at the inch opening on the left hand reflect yīn vacuity, this is [a disease of] the hand reverting yīn channel. The patient will suffer from palpitations, fear and unhappiness, pain in the heart and abdomen, difficulty in speaking, the heart as in a state of cold, and abstraction."

This is a preliminary description of the various manifestations and pathomechanisms involved in heart vacuity and repletion. Following this text, detailed descriptions of the pathomechanisms of heart repletion and heart vacuity are found in the *Zhū Bìng Yuán Hòu Lùn* ("Origin and Indicators of Disease"), *Shèng Jì Zǒng Lù* ("Sages' Salvation Records"), *Jì Shēng Fāng* (full name *Yán Shì Jì Shēng Fāng,* "Yan's Formulas for Saving

Lives"), *Dān Xī Shǒu Jìng* ("Dān-Xī's Hand Mirror"), and *Jǐng Yuè Quán Shū* ("Jǐng-Yuè's Complete Compendium").

Heart vacuity, mostly of such fundamental substances as heart qì, blood or fluids, tends to manifest as depletion damage in the organ functions related to heart qì, heart yáng, heart blood, and heart yīn. Heart repletion, mostly caused by the contraction of evil qì or the collection of pathological products, tends to adopt the pathomechanisms described as the struggle between right and evil qì.

In addition to this, the *Líng Shū* ("Magic Pivot") chapter "Visiting of Evil" contains the statement: "As for the evils that are located in the heart, they are all located in the pericardiac network." The *Wēn Rè Jīng Wěi* ("Warp and Weft of Warm Heat") chapter entitled "Yè Xiāng-Yán's External Contraction of Warmth and Heat" takes this idea one step further: "The heart is the great governor of the entire body and must not contract evil. If it contracts evil, the spirit leaves and the person will die. Whenever a statement refers to evil located in the heart, it is always the pericardiac network that has contracted it." This statement explicitly emphasizes that whenever external evils invade, they mostly attack the pericardiac network; it is only attributed to the heart when internal damage and vacuity damage cause a decline in function. There is no great value in debating whether heart diseases of repletion are definitely attributed to the pericardium and heart diseases of vacuity are definitely attributed to the heart. However, the significance of classifying the pathomechanisms of heart disease into vacuity and repletion can be determined with absolute certainty.

心病的病因，有外感六淫，特别是风、寒、湿、热之邪最易犯心。内伤七情，悲喜忧思，也易致心病。其它如禀赋不足，劳倦过度，饮食不节，嗜食肥甘，气机不畅，痰浊内阻，湿邪内停，水气上犯，瘀血停滞，久病重病，失治误治，以及其它脏腑疾病的传变，均可引起各种心的病变。

心的病机多以虚、实为纲，可分别反映心脏邪正双方的盛衰状态。从《素问•五藏生成篇》提出："思虑而伤心"开始，《黄帝内经》中已包含有"心虚"的论述。汉代华佗《中藏经》开始有专论心脏虚实寒热生死逆顺的篇章，提到"心气盛"、"心气实"、"心虚"等名称，从虚实盛衰的角度论及心病的病机变化。晋代王叔和的《脉经》更明确地阐述了"心实"和"心虚"的病机。如《平人迎神门气口前后脉篇》云："心实，左手寸口人迎以前脉阴实者，手厥阴经也。病苦闭，大便不利，腹满，四肢重，身热，苦胃胀；心虚，左手寸口人迎以前脉阴虚者，手厥阴经也。病苦悸恐不乐，心腹痛，难以言，心如寒状，恍惚。"初步描述了心的虚实病机变化时所引起的不同表现。其后，《诸病源候论》、《圣济总录》、《济生方》、《丹溪手镜》、《景岳全书》均有"心实"和"心虚"病机的详细论述。

心虚，主要由于心的气血津液等基本物质缺乏，易表现出心气、心阳、心血、心阴等脏腑功能的亏损；心实，多由感受邪气或病理产物停留，易呈现邪正相争的病机变化。

此外，《灵枢•邪客篇》有"邪之在于心者，皆在于心之包络"之说，《温热经纬•叶香岩外感温热篇》则进一步指出："心为一身之大主，而不受邪，受邪则神去而死。凡言邪之在心者，皆心之包络受之。"明确强调凡属外邪相侵，多侵犯心包络；内伤虚损，功能衰退，才归咎于心。至于是否一定要将心病偏实归咎于心包络，偏虚归属于心，并无多大争论价值。但有一点可以肯定，心病病机从虚、实分类确有十分重要的意义。

Literature Review

📖 *Zhōng Zàng Jīng* ("Central Treasury Canon"), Chapter on "Methods for Discussing Repletion and Vacuity, Cold and Heat, Life and Death, and Smoothness and Counterflow in the Heart Viscus"

"Exuberant heart qì causes dreams of happiness and laughter, worries and fear. Evil qì settling in the heart results in dreams of mountains and hills, smoke and fire. Heart distention causes shortness of breath, unquiet sleep, pain in the heart and abdomen, anguish…qì coming and going into the abdomen, heat with a liking for water, and drooling… Heart vacuity causes a fear of other people, closed eyes and a desire for sleep, a devitalized essence-spirit, and frenetic activity of the ethereal and corporeal souls. Replete heart qì causes inhibited urination, abdominal fullness, generalized heat and heaviness, seething with a desire to vomit ["seething" is an archaic expression that describes a subjective sensation of movement in the stomach], vomiting without any emission, rapid panting, and disquieted sleep. The pulse for this condition is a replete and large pulse at the left inch opening and at Man's Prognosis (*rén yíng*) [ST-9]. Heart vacuity leads to fear and susceptibility to fright, worry and unhappiness, pain in the chest and abdomen, trembling speech, aversion to cold and abstraction, a red face and yellow eyes, and a tendency to have spontaneous external bleeding. When examining the pulse, it is empty and faint at the inch opening both on the right and left."

This states that exuberance and debility of heart qì can cause pathological changes in the spirit-mind and the blood vessels.

📖 *Zhū Bìng Yuán Hòu Lùn* ("The Origin and Indicators of Disease"), "Symptoms of Heart Disease" and "Symptoms of Heart Suspension, Tension, Anguish, and Pain"

"Exuberance of heart qì refers to a superabundance of spirit. The person suffers from pain inside the chest, propping fullness in the rib-sides, pain below the rib-sides, pain between the anterior chest, back, arms, and armpit, pain on the inside of both arms, and incessant happiness and laughter. This is heart qì repletion and should therefore be treated by draining. Heart qì insufficiency causes an enlarged chest and abdomen, with pain stretching into the area below the rib-sides and into the lumbus and back, as well as fright palpitations and abstraction, lack of color, stiffness in the root of the tongue, and a tendency to experience anxiety and sorrow. All these symptoms are related to heart qì vacuity."

This states that heart qì exuberance is identical with heart repletion and heart qì insufficiency is identical with heart vacuity, and that one can distinguish between their respective pathomechanisms.

📖 *Qiān Jīn Yào Fāng* ("A Thousand Gold Pieces Prescriptions"), "Heart Repletion Heat"

"When the pulse at the inch opening on the left hand and in the front of Man's Prognosis (*rén yíng*) [ST-9] signifies yīn repletion, the hand lesser yīn channel is indicated. If the patient suffers from oppression, inhibited bowel movements, abdominal fullness, heaviness of the four limbs, and generalized heat effusion, it is called heart repletion heat."

This describes the pathomechanisms involved in heart repletion heat.

📖 *Qiān Jīn Yào Fāng* ("A Thousand Gold Pieces Prescriptions"), "Heart Vacuity Cold"

"When the pulses at the inch opening on the left hand and in the front of Man's Prognosis (*rén yíng*) [ST-9] are yīn and vacuous, this [is disease of] the hand lesser yīn channel. This is called heart vacuity cold if the patient suffers from palpitations, fear and unhappiness, pain in the heart and abdomen, difficulty in speaking, a heart as in a state of cold, and abstraction."

This describes the pathomechanisms involved in heart vacuity cold.

📖 *Shèng Jì Zǒng Lù* ("Sages' Salvation Records"), "Heart Vacuity"

"The condition of heart vacuity is marked by scant blood and debilitated qì, a yellow face, vexation and heat, a tendency to experience fear, palpitations, unhappiness, pain in the heart and abdomen, difficulty in speaking, intermittent emission of clear drool, distention and fullness in the heart and diaphragm, forgetfulness, a tendency to experience fright, dreaming and disturbed sleep, and abstraction of the essence-spirit. All

these symptoms are caused by vacuity cold in the hand lesser yīn channel. In the pulse, it is indicated by the observation of yīn vacuity at the
inch opening on the left hand and in the front of Man's Prognosis (*rén
yíng*) [ST-9]."

This further describes the pathomechanisms involved in heart vacuity
cold.

📖 *Shèng Jì Zǒng Lù* ("Sages' Salvation Records"), "Heart Repletion"

"When the pulse at the inch opening of the left hand before the bar is yīn
and replete, this is heart repletion. Qì ascends and there is fullness and
drum in the chest that spreads to the shoulders. Biǎn Què said that heart
repletion heat leads to panting counterflow, a full chest and breathing in
the supine position. The increase of heat in the hand lesser yīn channel
causes the disorder of heart repletion. Serious cases are marked by bitter-
ness in the mouth, intemperate drinking, and sores on the trunk and back.
This leads to pain of the thighs, knees, heels, and shins."

This further describes the pathomechanisms involved in heart repletion
heat.

📖 *Dān Xī Shǒu Jìng* ("Dān-Xī's Hand Mirror"), "Vacuity and
Repletion of the Five Viscera"

"The heart: Vacuity causes fulminant pain in the heart and abdomen, distention and fullness in the heart and diaphragm, intermittent spitting of
clear drool, excessive fright, fear, and abstraction, lack of color, stiffness
in the root of the tongue, and a floating and vacuous pulse. Repletion
causes vexation and derangement of the heart spirit, a red face, generalized heat, sores of the mouth and tongue, a dry throat, headache, heat in
the palms, spontaneous external bleeding, frequent laughing, and a pulse
that is surging and replete."

This is a more generalized description of the various clinical manifestations and pathomechanisms involved in heart vacuity and heart repletion.

文献评述

《中藏经•论心脏虚实寒热生死逆顺篇之法》说："心气盛，则梦
喜笑恐畏，邪气客于心，则梦山丘烟火。心胀则短气，夜卧不宁，
心腹痛，懊憹。... 气往来腹中，热喜水涎出。... 心虚则畏人，瞑目
欲眠，精神不依，魂魄妄乱。... 心气实则小便不利，腹满身热而
重，温温欲吐，吐而不出，喘息急，不安卧，其脉左寸口与人迎皆
实大者是也。心虚则恐惧多惊，忧思不乐，胸腹中苦痛，言语颤
栗，恶寒恍惚，面赤目黄，喜衄血，诊其脉，左右寸口两虚而微者
是也。"提出心气盛衰可引起神志和血脉病变。

《诸病源候论•心病候•心悬急懊痛候》说："心气盛，为神有余，则病胸内痛，胁支满，胁下痛，膺背膊腋间痛，两臂内痛，喜笑不休，是心气之实也，则宜泻之。心气不足，则胸腹大，胁下与腰背相引痛，惊悸恍惚，少颜色，舌本强，善忧悲，是为心气之虚也。"指出心气盛则是心实，心气不足则是心虚，可分别引起不同的病机变化。

《千金要方•心实热》说："左手寸口人迎以前脉阴实者，手少阴经也。病苦闭大便不利，腹满，四肢重，身热，名曰心实热也。"阐述了心实热引起的病机变化。

《千金要方•心虚寒》说："左手寸口人迎以前脉阴虚者，手少阴经也。病苦悸恐不乐，心腹痛，难以言，心如寒，恍惚，名曰心虚寒也。"阐述了心虚寒引起的病机变化。

《圣济总录•心虚》说："心虚之状，气血衰少，面黄烦热，多恐悸不乐，心腹痛难以言，时出清涎，心膈胀满，善忘多惊，梦寝不宁，精神恍惚，皆手少阴经虚寒所致。其脉见于左手寸口人迎以前阴虚者，乃其候也。"进一步阐述了心虚寒可引起的病机变化。

《圣济总录•心实》说："左手关前寸口阴实者，心实也。上气胸中满膨膨，与肩相引。扁鹊曰：心实热，则喘逆胸盈仰息，此手少阴为热所加，故为心实之病。甚则口苦引饮无度，体背生疮，以至股膝踹胫皆痛。"进一步阐述了心实热可引起的病机变化。

《丹溪手镜•五脏虚实》说："心：虚，心腹暴痛，心膈胀满，时唾清涎，多惊恐恍惚，少颜色，舌本强，脉浮虚。实，心神烦乱，面赤，身热，口舌生疮，咽燥，头痛，手心热，衄血，喜笑，脉洪实。"较为全面的论述了心虚、实病机变化时所引起的各种临床表现。

PART ONE

Pathomechanisms of Heart Repletion

心实的病机

Heart Repletion

The earliest descriptions of the pathomechanisms involved in heart repletion are found in the *Huáng Dì Nèi Jīng* ("The Yellow Emperor's Inner Canon"), in the *Sù Wèn* ("Plain Questions") chapter, "Methods of Treating Visceral Qì in Accordance with the Seasons." This example states: "Heart disorders cause pain in the chest, propping fullness in the rib-sides, pain below the rib-sides, pain between the anterior chest, the back, and the shoulder blades, and pain in the inside of both arms." In addition, it mentions the concepts of "heart qì repletion" and "heart qì heat," but it does not yet explicitly mention the term "heart repletion" as such.

It is not until the *Shèng Jì Zǒng Lù* ("Sages' Salvation Records") that the term "heart repletion" is mentioned specifically. As the "Section on the Heart Viscus" in this text states, "When the wrist pulse in the left hand before the bar reflects yīn repletion, this is a sign of heart repletion." Following this, the text *Jǐng Yuè Quán Shū* ("Jǐng-Yuè's Complete Compendium"), "Record of Faithful Transmission, Vacuity and Repletion" also states: "Heart repletion refers to excessive fire and excessive crying." All the above illustrate the historical existence of the pathomechanisms involved in heart repletion.

Disorders of heart repletion are predominantly caused by the contraction of external evils or by the collection of pathological products. Among externally contracted evils, fire, heat, cold, and dampness are the primary evils that invade the heart. The pathological products phlegm turbidity, damp turbidity, water-rheum, or static blood may collect and obstruct the heart vessels and heart spirit. Mutual binding of phlegm and fire may also harass the heart spirit. Additionally, the heart vessels may be obstructed by qì stagnation or blood stasis. To summarize, stasis of phlegm, dampness, fire, cold, and qì are the most important factors contributing to heart repletion.

The pathomechanisms of heart repletion can be differentiated into three major categories: heart repletion, heart repletion heat, and heart repletion cold. The differentiation depends on whether the condition tends towards neither cold nor heat, tends towards heat, or tends towards cold.

The pathomechanisms involved in heart repletion arise because qì stagnation, phlegm obstruction, damp encumbrance, water invasion, or blood stasis encumber and obstruct the heart viscus, leading to a violent struggle between evil and right. These are pathomechanisms of heart repletion, even when no prominent tendency towards cold or heat has yet appeared.

《黄帝内经》早有关于心实病机的论述，如《素问•藏气法时论》说："心病者，胸中痛，胁支满，胁下痛，膺背肩甲间痛，两臂内痛。"还提出"心气实"、"心气热"等概念，但未正式提出"心实"二字。直到《圣济总录》才正式提出"心实"的名称。如该书《心藏门》说"左手关前寸口脉阴实者，心实也。"后世《景岳全书•传忠录•虚实》亦说："心实者，多火而多哭。"均说明心实的病机客观存在。心病偏实主要因感受外邪或病理产物停留所致。感受外邪以火、热、寒、湿等病邪为主，侵犯心体；病理产物可为痰浊、湿浊、水饮、瘀血停留，闭阻心脉、心神。或为痰火互结，扰乱心神。或为气滞、血瘀、阻滞心脉。总之，痰、湿、火、寒、气、瘀是导致心实的主要因素。心实的病机根据不偏寒热、偏热、偏寒的不同，可分为心实、心实热、心实寒三个大类。

由于气滞、痰阻、湿困、水犯、血瘀等原因，困阻心脏，邪正之间剧烈相争，引起心实的病机变化，但还未出现明显偏寒或偏热的趋势，则为心实的病机。

Chapter One

Qì Stagnation Affecting the Heart

The heart governs the blood and vessels as well as the spirit-mind, predominantly through the activity of heart qì. Heart qì is not only the primary force in promoting the movement of blood, it also constitutes the material foundation for sustaining the activity of the heart spirit. The value of heart qì lies in its ceaseless movement; it should not pause or stagnate for even a single moment. If it is damaged by the seven affects (anxiety, thought, resentment, anger, sorrow, fright, and fear) and the qì dynamic is inhibited, heart qì becomes depressed. This results in pathological changes such as qì stagnation in the heart vessels or qì blocking the heart spirit.

气滞于心

心主血脉、神志，其中发挥主导作用的是心气。心气不仅是推动血液运行的动力，也是维持心神活动的物质基础。心气贵在周流不息，一刻不能停滞。忧思恨怒，悲愁惊恐，七情所伤，气机不畅，可使心气郁滞，进而引起气滞心脉或气闭心神等病变。

1.1 Qì Stagnating in the Heart Vessels

Emotional depression or long-term, sustained mental stimulus disturbs the state of the mind, causing emotional inhibition. This results in depression of heart qì. As the text *Zhèng Yīn Mài Zhì* ("Pathoconditions: Causes, Pulses, and Treatments"), "Heart Impediment," states, "A possible cause of heart impediment is found in anxiety, which taxes the heart and damages heart qì." This condition can be attributed to an impairment of the free-coursing function of the liver, causing binding depression of heart qì. If heart qì is unable to promote the movement of blood and the blood flow stagnates, there will be obstruction of the heart vessels. This manifests as intermittent stifling oppression, distention and pain in the chest with pain that stretches into the rib-sides, shoulder, and back, as well as frequent loud sighing. This type of heart pain is primarily associated with distention and is intimately connected to essence-spirit and affect-mind changes. It should be treated by coursing the liver and regulating qì while quickening blood and transforming stasis. To treat this, one may use Counterflow Cold Powder (*sì nì sǎn*) from the text *Shāng Hán Lùn* ("On Cold Damage"), with the addition of cyperus, unripe tangerine peel, curcuma, and peach kernel. This treatment focuses on moving qì and opening depression, with the secondary actions of quickening blood and transforming stasis.

Counterflow Cold Powder (四逆散 *sì nì sǎn*)

chái hú (柴胡 Bupleuri Radix, bupleurum)
bái sháo (白芍 Paeoniae Radix Alba, white peony)
zhǐ shí (枳实 Aurantii Fructus Immaturus, unripe bitter orange)
gān cǎo (甘草 Glycyrrhizae Radix, licorice)
Plus:
xiāng fù (香附 Cyperi Rhizoma, cyperus)
qīng pí (青皮 Citri Reticulatae Pericarpium Viride, unripe tangerine peel)
yù jīn (郁金 Curcumae Radix, curcuma)
táo rén (桃仁 Persicae Semen, peach kernel)
hóng huā (红花 Carthami Flos, carthamus)

气滞心脉

情志怫郁，或长期、持久的精神刺激，干扰心绪，心情不畅，而致心气郁滞。如《症因脉治·心痹》云："心痹之因，或焦虑劳心，心气受伤。"此为肝气不疏而致心气郁结，心气不能推动血行，血流滞塞，进而引起心脉痹阻。表现为心胸憋闷胀痛，牵引胸胁肩背而痛，时作时止，善太息。此种心痛以胀为主，与精神情志因素变化密切相关。治当疏肝理气，活血化瘀。可用《伤寒论》四逆散（柴胡、芍药、枳实、甘草）加香附、青皮、郁金、桃仁、红花，行气开郁为主，佐以活血化瘀进行调治。

Literature Review of Qì Stagnating in the Heart Vessels

📖 *Líng Shū* ("The Magic Pivot"), "Chapter on Oral Inquiry"

"Anxiety and thought make the heart ties tight. Tight heart ties cause the airways to be constrained. Constraint results in inhibition; therefore the patient sighs in order to stretch out."

This quotation points out that emotional disharmony restrains heart qì, causing oppression in the chest and sighing. Heart ties refer to the large blood vessels that communicate directly with the heart.

📖 *Zá Bìng Yuán Liú Xī Zhú* ("Incisive Light on the Source of Miscellaneous Disease"), "The Source of Heart Disease"

> "The seven affects are the cause of heart pain. … With the exception of joy, which dissipates qì to the outside, the others are all sufficient to cause binding depression of heart qì, giving rise to pain."

This quotation explains that the pathomechanism of qì stagnating in the heart vessels originates in the liver. From there, it influences the heart, causing qì stagnation and vessel impediment. When there is stoppage, there is heart pain.

文献评述

《灵枢·口问篇》说："忧思则心系急，心系急则气道约，约则不利，故太息以伸出之。"指出情志不调，约束心气，可致胸闷太息。

《杂病源流犀烛·心病源流》曰："七情之由作心痛。……除喜之气能散外，余皆足令心气郁结，而为痛也。"说明气滞心脉的病机发源于肝，影响于心，气滞而致脉痹，不通而作心痛。

1.2 Qì Blocking the Heart Spirit

Emotional excess may obstruct heart qì when a person is exposed to intense mental stimulation. This can be caused by frustration, anger, fright, or shock, or by encountering events such as damage, disease, or death, especially if the patient suffers from pain and sorrow to the point of wishing to die.

In mild cases, the lung qì will be blocked and depressed. This manifests in symptoms such as qì congestion in the chest, glomus, oppression, and constraint in the heart and chest, and hasty panting and rough breathing. The heart governs the spirit-mind and the heart qì is obstructed when the emotions are pushed to extremes. In turn, this influences the lung, inhibiting lung qì. When there is simultaneous obstruction of the qì dynamic of the heart and lung, qì collects in the chest and ascends counterflow. This condition should be treated by moving qì, opening impediment, downbearing qì, and calming panting. For treatment, one may use a modified version of Tangerine Peel, Unripe Bitter Orange, and Fresh Ginger Decoction (*jú pí zhǐ shí shēng jiāng tāng*) from the *Jīn Guì Yào Lüè* ("Essential Prescriptions of the Golden Coffer"), "Chapter on Chest Impediment, Heart Pain, and Shortness of Breath."

Tangerine Peel, Unripe Bitter Orange, and Fresh Ginger Decoction (橘皮枳实生姜汤 *jú pí zhǐ shí shēng jiāng tāng*)
jú pí (橘皮 Citri Reticulatae Pericarpium, tangerine peel) *zhǐ shí* (枳实 Aurantii Fructus Immaturus, unripe bitter orange) *shēng jiāng* (生姜 Zingiberis Rhizoma Recens, fresh ginger)

In severe cases, there will be chaotic counterflow of qì and blood that clouds the orifices of the heart. The heart will be unable to govern the spirit-mind, and the heart spirit will float astray, resulting in sudden clouding collapse, an unclear spirit-mind, and loss of consciousness. This condition should be treated by coursing the liver, rectifying qì, and opening the orifices with aromatic medicinals. For a formula, one may use a modified form of Storax Pill (*sū hé xiāng wán*) from the *Tài Píng Huì Mín Hé Jì Jú Fāng* ("Tài-Píng Imperial Grace Pharmacy Formulas").

Storax Pill (苏合香丸 *sū hé xiāng wán*)
sū hé xiāng (苏合香 Styrax, storax) *rǔ xiāng* (乳香 Olibanum, frankincense) *shè xiāng* (麝香 Moschus, musk) *dīng xiāng* (丁香 Caryophylli Flos, clove) *chén xiāng* (沉香 Aquilariae Lignum Resinatum, aquilaria) *ān xī xiāng* (安息香 Benzoinum, benzoin) *tán xiāng* (檀香 Santali Albi Lignum, sandalwood) *mù xiāng* (木香 Aucklandiae Radix, costusroot) [*chǎo*] *xiāng fù* ([炒]香附 Cyperi Rhizoma, cyperus [stir-fried]) *bái zhú* (白术 Atractylodis Macrocephalae Rhizoma, white atractylodes) *bì bō* (荜茇 Piperis Longi Fructus, long pepper) *hē zǐ* (诃子 Chebulae Fructus, chebule) *zhū shā* (朱砂 Cinnabaris, cinnabar) *xī jiǎo* (犀角 Rhinocerotis Cornu, rhinoceros horn) *bīng piàn* (冰片 Borneolum, borneol)

气闭心神

如果受到强烈的精神刺激，或恼怒惊骇，或遇伤残病死等事，悲痛欲绝，情志过极，遏阻心气，轻则闭郁肺气，可见胸中气塞、心胸痞闷不舒、喘促气粗等症。这是由于心主神志，情志过极，心气被遏，进而影响肺气不利，心肺气机同时阻滞，气停胸中，上逆而成。治宜行气开痹，降气平喘，可用《金匮要略•胸痹心痛短气篇》<u>橘皮枳实生姜汤</u>（橘皮、枳实、生姜）加减治疗。重则气血逆乱，蒙闭心窍，心不主神志，心神浮越，而致突然昏倒，神志不清，不省人事。治宜疏肝理气，芳香开窍，方用《太平惠民和剂局方》<u>苏合香丸</u>（苏合香油、熏陆香、麝香、丁香、沉香、安息香、檀香、青木香、炒香附、白术、荜拨、煨柯子、朱砂、犀角、冰片）加减。

Literature Review of Qì Blocking the Heart Spirit

📖 *Jǐng Yuè Quán Shū* ("Jǐng-Yuè's Complete Compendium"), "Schema of Miscellaneous Patterns, Reverse Flow"

"The condition of qì repletion and reversal manifests with qì indignation and bad temper. The pulse will be sunken, string-like, and slippery, with panting and fullness in the chest and diaphragm. This is a pattern of qì counterflow."

This quote refers to the pattern of qì reversal and repletion, which is formed because of a depressed and blocked qì dynamic. It is closely related to heart qì depression. The panting and fullness of the chest and diaphragm are linked to depressed qì damaging the liver and heart. Liver and heart qì stagnation causes impaired depurative downbearing of the lung, resulting in ascendant counterflow of lung qì. Sudden collapse, an unclear spirit-mind, and clouding and fretting of the heart spirit are symptoms that never appear unless the heart orifices are clouded and blocked.

This quotation explains that when the heart is subjected to intense mental stimulation, there may be sudden block and chaotic counterflow of the heart qì. This causes the heart spirit to lose its ability to govern, leading to clouding collapse.

文献评述

《景岳全书•杂证谟•厥逆》说："气实而厥者，其形气愤然勃然，脉沉弦而滑，胸膈喘满，此气逆证也。"此乃气机郁闭而成的气厥实证，与心气郁滞有密切的关系。胸膈喘满，为气郁伤肝损心，肝心气滞，肺失肃降，肺气上逆所致；卒然倒仆，神志不清，心神昏愦，非心窍蒙闭，绝不可见。说明心因受到强烈精神刺激，心气陡然闭塞逆乱，进而心神失主，方能导致昏仆。

Summary of Qì Stagnation Affecting the Heart

1. Qì Stagnating in the Heart Vessels
   Obstruction of the heart vessels: Intermittent stifling oppression, distention, and pain in the heart and chest, with pain that stretches into the chest, rib-sides, shoulder, and back, accompanied by frequent sighing
2. Qì Blocking the Heart Spirit
   Mild cases: Qì congestion in the chest, glomus and constraint in the chest, hasty panting and rough breathing
   Severe cases: Chaotic counterflow of qì and blood, an ungoverned heart spirit, sudden clouding collapse, and an unclear spirit-mind

气滞于心

气滞心脉
    心脉痹阻 —— 心胸憋闷胀痛，牵引胸胁肩背，时作时止，善太息。
气闭心神
    轻者 —— 胸中气塞、胸痞不舒、喘促气粗。
    重者 —— 气血逆乱，心神无主，突然昏倒，神志不清。

Chapter Two

Phlegm Obstructing the Heart

Phlegm turbidity is a pathological product that is formed when a fluid disorder causes fluids to collect in the inner body. Phlegm turbidity collecting in the inner body obstructs heart qì; it may impede the heart vessels or cloud and block the heart spirit.

痰阻于心

痰浊是津液失调停于体内而形成的病理产物，痰浊内停，阻滞心气，既可痹阻心脉，又可蒙闭心神。

2.1 Phlegm Obstructing the Heart Vessels

In a person with constitutional obesity or an internal exuberance of phlegm-dampness, the chronic lingering of phlegm turbidity evil places added strain on heart qì. Phlegm turbidity is sticky, stagnating, and difficult to move, so it can cause heart qì to become drowsy and depressed. This inhibits the qì dynamic and slows the movement of heart blood, causing gradual obstruction of the heart vessels. It can manifest in pathoconditions that feature stifling oppression and pain in the heart and chest, or heart palpitations and shortness of breath. Moreover, since phlegm turbidity collects inside the body, it can manifest with accompanying symptoms such as obesity, a heavy cumbersome body, and thick slimy tongue fur.

This condition should be treated by eliminating phlegm and opening impediment. One should choose the formula Trichosanthes, Chinese Chive, and Pinellia Decoction (*guā lóu xiè bái bàn xià tāng*) from the *Jīn Guì Yào Lüè* ("Essential Prescriptions of the Golden Coffer").

Trichosanthes, Chinese Chive, and Pinellia Decoction
(栝楼薤白半夏汤 *guā lóu xiè bái bàn xià tāng*)

---

guā lóu (瓜蒌 Trichosanthis Fructus, trichosanthes)
xiè bái (薤白 Allii Macrostemonis Bulbus, Chinese chive)

bàn xià (半夏 Pinelliae Rhizoma, pinellia)
bái jiǔ (白酒 Granorum Spiritus Incolor, white liquor)

The *Jīn Guì Yào Lüè* ("Essential Prescriptions of the Golden Coffer"), "Chapter on Disorders of Chest Impediment, Heart Pain, and Shortness of Breath" states, "In cases of chest impediment with an inability to sleep and heart pain stretching through to the back, Trichosanthes, Chinese Chive, and Pinellia Decoction (*guā lóu xiè bái bàn xià tāng*) governs."

A commentary in the *Jīn Guì Yào Lüè Xīn Diǎn* ("Commentary on Essential Prescriptions of the Golden Coffer") states, "Chest impediment with an inability to sleep is due to lung qì rising and failing to descend. Heart pain stretching through to the back is due to congestion and disharmony of heart qì; this is a serious impediment condition. The condition is aggravated by phlegm-rheum; therefore, one should add pinellia (*bàn xià*) to the chest impediment prescription in order to expel phlegm-rheum."

These quotations expound in detail the pathomechanism of phlegm turbidity congesting the heart and lung qì, resulting in obstruction of the heart vessels.

痰阻心脉

素体肥胖，或痰湿内盛之人，因痰浊之邪久恋，粘滞难行，增加心气阻力，可使心气困顿而郁滞。气机不畅，心血运迟，渐致心脉痹阻。可见心胸憋闷疼痛，心悸气短等症，并因痰湿停留体内，而兼见形体肥胖，身体困重，舌苔厚腻。

治宜除痰开痹，方剂可选《金匮要略》栝蒌薤白半夏汤（栝蒌实、薤白、半夏、白酒）。如《金匮要略•胸痹心痛短气病篇》曰："胸痹不得卧，心痛彻背者，栝蒌薤白半夏汤主之。"《金匮要略心典》在注释时云："胸痹不得卧，是肺气上而不下也；心痛彻背，是心气塞而不和也，其痹为尤甚矣。所以然者，有痰饮以为之援也，故胸痹药中加半夏以逐痰饮。"详细阐明了痰浊壅塞心肺之气而致心脉痹阻的病机.

Literature Review of Phlegm Obstructing the Heart Vessels

📖 *Zhèng Yīn Mài Zhì* ("Pathoconditions: Causes, Pulses, and Treatments"), "Chest Impediment"

"The causes of chest impediment include dietary irregularities, damage by hunger and satiety, congealed phlegm and stagnant blood, and turbidity in the center burner. These factors cause the pathoconditions of food blockage, oppression, and pain."

This quotation points out that an internal collection of phlegm-turbidity may cause congealed phlegm and blood stagnation, which can obstruct the heart vessels.

> ### 文献评述
>
> 《症因脉治•胸痹》说："胸痹之因，饮食不节，饥饱损伤，痰凝血滞，中焦混浊，则闭食闷痛之症作矣。"指出痰浊内停，痰凝血滞，可闭阻心脉。

2.2 Phlegm Clouding the Heart Spirit

Heart qì is one of the material foundations for supporting the activities of the spirit-mind. Phlegm turbidity that has collected internally may follow the qì dynamic to ascend counterflow and cloud the orifices of the heart. This impedes the material supply of heart qì for the activities of the spirit-mind and deprives the heart spirit of nourishment. When the spirit-light fails to govern, the result is a confounded and deranged essence-spirit and an unclear spirit-mind. The pathological manifestations of phlegm obstructing the heart orifices vary, owing to differences in causation.

If liver qì depression inhibits movement of the qì dynamic, gathering depression may engender phlegm. This causes obstruction of heart qì, clouding of the heart orifices, and mental derangement; the main result is deep quietude. This pattern mostly manifests as depression and unhappiness, an indifferent expression, muttering to oneself, rambling and incoherent speech, and dullness of the spirit-mind; it leads to feeble-mindedness and withdrawal. This condition should be treated by coursing the liver and opening depression while sweeping phlegm and opening the orifices. For a formula, choose Free Wanderer Powder (*xiāo yáo sǎn*) from the text *Tài Píng Huì Mín Hé Jì Jú Fāng* ("Tài-Píng Imperial Grace Pharmacy Formulas"), combined with Phlegm-Abducting Decoction (*dǎo tán tāng*) from *Jì Shēng Fāng* (full name *Yán Shì Jì Shēng Fāng* ("Yan's Formulas for Saving Lives")).

Free Wanderer Powder (逍遥散 *xiāo yáo sǎn*)
chái hú (柴胡 Bupleuri Radix, bupleurum)
dāng guī (当归 Angelicae Sinensis Radix, Chinese angelica)
bái sháo (白芍 Paeoniae Radix Alba, white peony)
bái zhú (白术 Atractylodis Macrocephalae Rhizoma, white atractylodes)
fú líng (茯苓 Poria, poria)
bò hé (薄荷 Menthae Herba, mint)
gān cǎo (甘草 Glycyrrhizae Radix, licorice)

Phlegm-Abducting Decoction (导痰汤 *dǎo tán tāng*)

nán xīng (南星 Arisaematis Rhizoma, arisaema)

bàn xià (半夏 Pinelliae Rhizoma, pinellia)

chén pí (陈皮 Citri Reticulatae Pericarpium, tangerine peel)

fú líng (茯苓 Poria, poria)

zhǐ shí (枳实 Aurantii Fructus Immaturus, unripe bitter orange)

gān cǎo (甘草 Glycyrrhizae Radix, licorice)

If a person has a constitutional tendency to accumulate hidden phlegm internally, sudden fright or excessive taxation fatigue can cause irregularities in the qì dynamic of the bowels and viscera. This will trigger the accumulation of phlegm. Phlegm and qì contending with each other may cloud the orifices of the heart and induce stirring of liver wind.

If liver wind is complicated by phlegm, it may harass internally. The phlegm blocks the heart spirit, resulting in sudden collapse and immediate unconsciousness. When liver wind stirs internally, there are signs such as convulsions of the extremities, a clenched jaw, and upward staring eyes. When phlegm qì is forced upward, there will be drool foaming at the mouth and utterance of all sorts of sounds; this is a symptom of epilepsy. It should be treated by calming the liver and extinguishing wind while flushing phlegm and opening the orifices. For a formula, use a modified version of Fit-Settling Pill (*dìng xián wán*) from Héng Guó-Péng's *Medical Insights*.

Fit-Settling Pill (定痫丸 *dìng xián wán*)

tiān má (天麻 Gastrodiae Rhizoma, gastrodia)

quán xiē (全蝎 Scorpio, scorpion)

jiāng cán (僵蚕 Bombyx Batryticatus, silkworm)

chuān bèi mǔ (川贝母 Fritillariae Cirrhosae Bulbus, Sìchuān fritillaria)

dǎn xīng (胆星 Arisaema cum Bile, bile arisaema)

bàn xià (半夏 Pinelliae Rhizoma, pinellia)

zhú lì (竹沥 Bambusae Succus, bamboo sap)

shí chāng pú (石菖蒲 Acori Tatarinowii Rhizoma, acorus)

hǔ pò (琥珀 Succinum, amber)

fú shén (茯神 Poria cum Pini Radice, root poria)

yuǎn zhì (远志 Polygalae Radix, polygala)

zhū shā (朱砂 Cinnabaris, cinnabar)

fú líng (茯苓 Poria, poria)

chén pí (陈皮 Citri Reticulatae Pericarpium, tangerine peel)

dān shēn (丹参 Salviae Miltiorrhizae Radix, salvia)

mài dōng (麦冬 Ophiopogonis Radix, ophiopogon)
shēng jiāng zhī (姜汁 Zingiberis Rhizomatis Succus, ginger juice)
gān cǎo (甘草 Glycyrrhizae Radix, licorice)

If a person has a constitutional tendency to experience ascendant hyperactivity of liver yáng, yáng becomes hyperactive and unrestrained, causing liver wind to spin internally. Phlegm turbidity will follow the wind and yáng upwards, clouding the heart orifices and causing sudden loss of the heart spirit. This can cause abrupt clouding of the spirit with sudden collapse. Phlegm-drool and wind may gush into the throat, resulting in a stiff tongue, sluggish speech and phlegm rale in the throat. When phlegm and drool penetrate transversely into the channels and vessels, it is also possible to observe deviated eyes and mouth and hemiplegia, which occur as secondary symptoms of wind strike. This condition should be treated by flushing phlegm and opening the orifices while coursing wind and freeing the network vessels. Ordinarily, choose modified versions of Phlegm-Flushing Decoction (*dí tán tāng*) from the *Qī Xiào Liáng Fāng* ("Extraordinarily Effective Formulas"), in combination with Pull Aright Powder (*qiān zhèng sǎn*) from *Yáng Shì Jiā Cáng Fāng* ("Yáng's Family Heritage Formulas").

Phlegm-Flushing Decoction (涤痰汤 *dí tán tāng*)

nán xīng (南星 Arisaematis Rhizoma, arisaema)
bàn xià (半夏 Pinelliae Rhizoma, pinellia)
fú líng (茯苓 Poria, poria)
jú hóng (橘红 Citri Reticulatae Pericarpium Rubrum, red tangerine peel)
zhǐ shí (枳实 Aurantii Fructus Immaturus, unripe bitter orange)
zhú rú (竹茹 Bumbusae Caulis in Taenia, bamboo shavings)
rén shēn (人参 Ginseng Radix, ginseng)
shí chāng pú (石菖蒲 Acori Tatarinowii Rhizoma, acorus)
shēng jiāng (生姜 Zingiberis Rhizoma Recens, fresh ginger)
gān cǎo (甘草 Glycyrrhizae Radix, licorice)

Pull Aright Powder (牵正散 *qiān zhèng sǎn*)

bái fù zǐ (白附子 Typhonii Gigantei Rhizoma, giant typhonium rhizome)
jiāng cán (僵蚕 Bombyx Batryticatus, silkworm)
quán xiē (全蝎 Scorpio, scorpion)

To summarize, the heart spirit fails to govern when blocked and clouded by phlegm turbidity. This gives rise to the pathomechanisms involved in withdrawal, epilepsy, feeble-mindedness, and many other mental irregularities.

蒙闭心神

心气是维系神志活动的物质基础之一。痰浊内停，随气机上逆，蒙蔽心窍，阻碍心气对神志活动的物质供给，心神失养，神明失主，而致精神迷乱，神志不清。痰阻心窍，随其原因不同，病理表现各有差异。若为肝气郁滞，气机流行不畅，郁聚生痰，心气被阻，心窍蒙蔽，精神错乱多以沉静为主。其证多见抑郁不乐，表情淡漠，喃喃自语，语无伦次，神志呆滞，发为痴癫。治宜疏肝开郁，豁痰开窍。方选《太平惠民和剂局方》逍遥散（柴胡、当归、白芍、白术、茯苓、薄荷、甘草）合《济生方》导痰汤（南星、半夏、茯苓、陈皮、枳实、甘草）。

若平素积痰内伏，突受惊恐或劳倦过度，脏腑气机失调，触动积痰，痰气互相搏击，蒙蔽心窍，引动肝风。肝风挟痰内扰，痰闭心神，则卒然倒仆，瞬息不省人事。肝风内动，则见手足抽搐、牙关紧闭、两目上视；痰气上迫，则口吐涎沫、发出各种叫声，则为痫证。治宜平肝熄风，涤痰开窍，方用程国彭《医学心悟》定痫丸（天麻、全蝎、僵蚕、川贝、胆星、半夏、竹沥、石菖蒲、琥珀、茯神、远志、辰砂、茯苓、陈皮、丹参、麦冬、姜汁、甘草）加减。

若素体肝阳上亢，阳亢无制，肝风内旋，痰浊随风阳上升，蒙塞心窍，心神顿失，亦可卒发神昏，突然倒仆。痰涎风涌咽喉，可致舌强语謇、喉中痰鸣，痰涎横窜经脉而见口眼歪斜、半身不遂、发为中风后遗症。治宜涤痰开窍，疏风通络。常选《奇效良方》涤痰汤（制南星、制半夏、茯苓、橘红、枳实、竹茹、人参、石菖蒲、生姜、甘草）合《杨氏家藏方》牵正散（白附子、僵蚕、全蝎）加减。总之，痰浊蒙闭，心神失主，可引起癫、痫、痴、呆多种精神失常的病机变化。

Literature Review of Phlegm Clouding the Heart Spirit

📖 *Jǐng Yuè Quán Shū* ("Jǐng-Yuè's Complete Compendium"), "Schema of Miscellaneous Patterns: Mania, Withdrawal, and Feeble-mindedness"

"All cases of qì counterflow and phlegm stagnation can congest the channels and network vessels, congesting the orifices of the heart."

This quotation points out that depression of the qì dynamic causes non-distribution of fluids. This leads to the formation of phlegm, which can cloud and block the orifices of the heart.

📖 *Lín Zhèng Zhǐ Nán Yī Àn* ("A Clinical Guide with Case Histories"), "Section on Withdrawal and Epilepsy"

> "Withdrawal is caused by the accumulation of anxiety and depression. The disease is located in the heart, spleen, and pericardium. The three yīn channels become covered and fail to diffuse; therefore qì is depressed, leading to confounding phlegm. This causes the spirit-mind to become confused."

This quotation points out that qì depression generates phlegm, which clouds and blocks the heart spirit. This causes the spirit-mind to become deranged and leads to the onset of withdrawal disorders.

📖 *Biàn Zhèng Lù* ("Record of Pattern Identification"), "Section on Feeble-mindedness"

> "The formation of feeble-mindedness invariably has a cause. Most likely, the initial stage originates in liver qì depression. The final stages are caused by the debilitation of stomach qì. When the liver is depressed, wood restrains earth and phlegm fails to be transformed. Stomach debility results in earth failing to dam water and non-dispersion of phlegm. Because of this, phlegm accumulates in the center of the chest, lingering in the area outside the heart. It causes the spirit-light to be unclear, thereby generating the disorder of feeble-mindedness."

This quotation elaborates on the pathomechanism by which liver qì depression, complicated by phlegm, clouds the heart spirit. The result is feeble-mindedness and withdrawal.

📖 *Lín Zhèng Zhǐ Nán Yī Àn* ("A Clinical Guide with Case Histories"), "Section on Withdrawal and Epilepsy"

> "The pattern of epilepsy is caused either by fright and fear, dietary irregularities, or fright contracted in the fetal stage. These can cause unstable visceral qì and enduring irregularities. Once triggered by accumulated phlegm, reversal of qì and internal wind arise suddenly in conjunction with violent counterflow. Nothing can stop this; one can merely wait until the qì returns by itself to its proper flow."

This describes how liver wind with phlegm can cloud the heart spirit and cause qì and blood to counterflow chaotically, resulting in an epilepsy pattern.

📖 *Zhāng Shì Yī Tōng* ("Zhang's Clear View of Medicine"), "Epilepsy"

> "Liver wind is the only cause of convulsions. In cases of convulsions, the fat and humors that flow around the body are forced to ascend. They follow the counterflow qì and are expelled from the mouth."

This quotation points out that liver wind, in conjunction with phlegm clouding the heart spirit, can lead to an epilepsy pattern.

📖 *Dān Xī Xīn Fǎ* ("Dān-Xī's Heart-Approach"), "Wind Strike"

> "Wind strike is mainly attributed to blood vacuity and the presence of phlegm; the phlegm should be treated first and the blood should be nourished and moved later on. It is possible that the vacuity exists in conjunction with fire (sometimes regarded as phlegm) and dampness. ... Hemiplegia is mostly caused by excess phlegm."

This quotation explains that liver yáng transforms into wind. Wind and phlegm may obstruct the network vessels, resulting in hemiplegia.

文献评述

《景岳全书•杂证谟•癫狂痴呆》说："凡气有所逆，痰有所滞，皆能壅闭经络，格塞心窍。"指出气机郁滞，津液失布，化生痰液，可蒙闭心窍。

《临证指南医案•癫痫门》说："癫由积忧积郁，病在心、脾、包络，三阴蔽而不宣，故气郁则痰迷，神志为之混淆。"指出气郁生痰，蒙闭心神，使神志紊乱，发为癫病。

《辨证录•呆病门》说："呆病之成，必有其因。大约其始也，起于肝气之郁；其终也，由于胃气之衰。肝郁则木克土，而痰不能化；胃衰则土不制水而痰不能消，于是痰积于胸中，盘踞心外，使神明不清，而成呆病矣。"精辟地阐述肝气挟痰，蒙蔽心神而成痴癫的病机。

《临证指南医案•癫痫门》说："痫证或因惊恐，或由饮食不节，或由母腹中受惊，以致脏气不平，经久失调，一触积痰，厥气内风，卒焉暴逆，莫能禁止，待其气反然后已。"阐述了肝风夹痰，蒙闭心神，气血逆乱，引起痫证的病机。

《张氏医通•痫》说："惟有肝风故作搐搦，搐搦则通身之脂液逼迫而上，随逆气而吐出于口也。"指出肝风夹痰，蒙闭心神，可致痫证。

《丹溪心法•中风》说："中风大率主血虚有痰，治痰为先，次养血行血。或属虚挟火（一作痰）与湿。…半身不遂，大率多痰。"说明肝阳化风，风痰阻络，可致半身不遂。

Summary of Phlegm Obstructing the Heart

1. Phlegm Obstructing the Heart Vessels

   Heart vessel obstruction: Stifling oppression and pain in the heart and chest, heart palpitations and shortness of breath, obesity, a heavy cumbersome body, thick slimy tongue fur

2. Phlegm Clouding the Heart Spirit

   Liver qì complicated by phlegm: Depression and unhappiness, indifferent expression, muttering to oneself, incoherent speech, dullness of the spirit-mind, onset of feeble-mindedness and withdrawal

   Liver wind complicated by phlegm: Sudden collapse with unconsciousness, convulsions in the hands and feet, a clenched jaw, upturned eyes, drool foaming at the mouth, and utterance of a variety of sounds

   Liver yáng transforming into wind: Sudden onset of clouded spirit with sudden collapse, a stiff tongue and sluggish speech, phlegm rale in the throat, deviation of the mouth and eyes, and hemiplegia

痰阻于心

痰阻心脉:

心脉痹阻 —— 心胸憋闷疼痛，心悸气短，形体肥胖，身体困重，舌苔厚腻。

痰蒙心神

肝气夹痰 —— 抑郁不乐，表情淡漠，喃喃自语，语无伦次，神志呆滞，发为痴癫。

肝风夹痰 —— 卒然倒仆，不省人事。手足抽搐、牙关紧闭、两目上视；口吐涎沫、发出各种叫声。

肝阳化风 —— 卒发神昏，突然倒仆。舌强语謇、喉中痰鸣，口眼歪斜、半身不遂。

Chapter Three

Dampness Encumbering the Heart

"Dampness encumbering the heart" refers to dampness that ascends to invade the heart. It is caused by either externally contracted water-damp evil or an internal collection of damp turbidity from the spleen's failure to fortify and move. Both causes are involved in the pathomechanisms of damp turbidity encumbering the heart vessels and the heart spirit.

湿困于心

外感水湿之邪，或脾失健运而湿浊内停，上犯于心，均可引起湿浊之邪困阻心脉和心神的病机。

3.1 Dampness Encumbering the Heart Vessels

Externally contracted wind-damp evils invade the channels in the exterior as well as the joints of the whole body. Evils trap and depress defensive yáng and impede the flow of channel qì. This can result in aversion to cold and heat effusion, headache and generalized pain, and swollen painful joints.

If external dampness advances further to invade the heart viscus or if internally engendered damp evil ascends to invade the heart, the heart vessels will be encumbered and blocked and heart qì will be impeded. Heart qì will lack the power to move the blood and will compensate with heart throbbing and an accelerated heartbeat. This will cause heart palpitations, fearful throbbing, and exhaustion of the heart with panting, oppression in the chest, and shortness of breath.

When damp evil obstructs the heart vessels and impedes the movement of blood to cause qì and blood stagnation, it manifests in a soot-black facial complexion, a darkened tongue, and the presence of stasis macules and stasis speckles. Although the pathomechanism of heart qì vacuity may be concurrently observed, the nature of this disorder is categorized as a repletion pattern because it is caused by the collection of evil qì or damp evil, a pathological product. It should be treated by coursing wind and eliminating dampness while freeing the vessels and diffusing the impediment. The formula Fangji and Astragalus Decoction (*fáng jǐ huáng qí tāng*) from the *Jīn Guì Yào Lüe* ("Essential Prescriptions of the Golden Coffer") is often used to treat this disorder.

Fangji and Astragalus Decoction (防己黄芪汤 *fáng jǐ huáng qí tāng*)

fáng jǐ (防己 Stephaniae Tetrandrae Radix, fangji)
huáng qí (黄芪 Astragali Radix, astragalus)
bái zhú (白朮 Atractylodis Macrocephalae Rhizoma, white atractylodes)
gān cǎo (甘草 Glycyrrhizae Radix, licorice)
Plus:
guì zhī (桂枝 Cinnamomi Ramulus, cinnamon twig)
chì sháo (赤芍 Paeoniae Radix Rubra, red peony)
chuān xiōng (川芎 Chuanxiong Rhizoma, chuanxiong)
jī xuè téng (鸡血藤 Spatholobi Caulis, spatholobus)

湿困心脉

外感风湿之邪，侵犯体表经脉、周身关节，遏郁卫阳，阻碍经气，可致恶寒发热，头身疼痛，关节肿痛。外湿进一步侵犯心脏，或内生湿邪上犯于心，则可困阻心脉，阻碍心气，心气推动运血无力，代偿性出现心跳加快，则为心悸怔忡，心累气喘，胸闷短气。

　　湿邪困阻心脉，阻碍血行，气血瘀滞，可致面色黧黑，舌质晦暗，有瘀斑、瘀点。由于有致病邪气和病理产物湿邪的停留，虽然伴见心气虚的病机，病性仍属实证。治宜疏风除湿，通脉宣痹。常用《金匮要略》<u>防己黄芪汤</u>（防己、黄芪、白术、甘草）加桂枝、赤芍、川芎、鸡血藤进行治疗。

3.2 Dampness Encumbering the Heart Spirit

When damp evils invade the heart, yīn dampness spreads and impedes heart qì. This deprives the heart spirit of the nourishment of qì and blood, preventing it from executing its activating and vitalizing functions. In mild cases, the person's mental state will be drowsy, leading to somnolence and excessive sleeping. In severe cases, damp turbidity will form phlegm that will cloud the heart spirit, leading to abstraction, drowsiness, and even stupor or unconsciousness. It should be treated by eliminating dampness and discharging turbidity while opening the orifices with aroma. For a formula, use Storax Pill (*sū hé xiāng wán*) from the text *Tài*

Píng Huì Mín Hé Jì Jú Fāng ("Tài-Píng Imperial Grace Pharmacy Formulas") or Jade Pivot Elixir (*yù shū dān*) from the *Piàn Yù Xīn Shū* ("A Piece of Jade-like Understandings").

Storax Pill (苏合香丸 *sū hé xiāng wán*)
sū hé xiāng (苏合香 Styrax, storax)
rǔ xiāng (乳香 Olibanum, frankincense)
shè xiāng (麝香 Moschus, musk)
dīng xiāng (丁香 Caryophylli Flos, clove)
chén xiāng (沉香 Aquilariae Lignum Resinatum, aquilaria)
ān xī xiāng (安息香 Benzoinum, benzoin)
tán xiāng (檀香 Santali Albi Lignum, sandalwood)
mù xiāng (木香 Aucklandiae Radix, costusroot)
(*chǎo*) *xiāng fù* ([炒]香附 Cyperi Rhizoma, cyperus [stir-fried])
bái zhú (白术 Atractylodis Macrocephalae Rhizoma, white atractylodes)
bì bō (荜茇 Piperis Longi Fructus, long pepper)
hē zǐ (诃子 Chebulae Fructus, chebule)
zhū shā (朱砂 Cinnabaris, cinnabar)
xī jiǎo (犀角 Rhinocerotis Cornu, rhinoceros horn)
bīng piàn (冰片 Borneolum, borneol)

Jade Pivot Elixir (玉枢丹 *yù shū dān*)
shān cí gū (山慈姑 Cremastrae seu Pleiones Pseudobulbus, cremastra/pleione [pseudobulb])
shè xiāng (麝香 Moschus, musk)
qiān jīn zǐ shuāng (千金子霜 Euphorbiae Semen Pulveratum, caper spurge seed frost)
dà jǐ (大戟 Euphorbiae seu Knoxiae Radix, euphorbia/knoxia)
wǔ bèi zǐ (五倍子 Galla Chinensis Galla, sumac gallnut)
xióng huáng (雄黄 Realgar, realgar)
zhū shā (朱砂 Cinnabaris, cinnabar)

湿困心神

湿邪犯心，阴湿弥漫，阻碍心气，使心神失却气血的濡养，不能发挥激发、振奋作用，轻者使人神情困顿，引起嗜睡多眠。重者湿浊酿痰，蒙闭心神，导致恍惚、朦胧，甚至神志昏迷，不省人事，出现一派危重局面。治宜除湿泄浊，芳香开窍。方用《太平惠民和剂局方》苏合香丸或《片玉新书》玉枢丹（山慈菇、麝香、千金子霜、红芽大戟、五倍子、雄黄、朱砂）。

Summary of Dampness Encumbering the Heart

1. Dampness Encumbering the Heart Vessels

   Damp evil invading the exterior: Aversion to cold and heat effusion, headache and generalized pain, swollen and painful joints

   Dampness encumbering the heart qi: Heart palpitations, fearful throbbing, and exhaustion of the heart with panting, oppression in the chest and shortness of breath

   Dampness encumbering the blood vessels: Soot-black complexion, darkened tongue, stasis macules and stasis speckles

2. Dampness Encumbering the Heart Spirit

   Mild cases: Drowsy mental state, somnolence and excessive sleeping

   Severe cases: Abstraction and drowsiness with stupor or unconsciousness

---

湿困于心：

湿困心脉

    湿邪犯表 —— 恶寒发热，头身疼痛，关节肿痛。

    湿困心气 —— 心悸怔忡，心累气喘，胸闷短气。

    湿困血脉 —— 面色黧黑，舌质晦暗，瘀斑瘀点。

湿困心脉

    轻者 —— 神情困顿，嗜睡多眠。

    重者 —— 恍惚朦胧，神志昏迷，不省人事。

Chapter Four

Water Invading the Heart

The two main components of blood are construction qì and fluids. The heart governs the blood vessels and heart qì simultaneously propels the movement of both blood and fluids. When heart qì is vacuous and weak, it is unable to move the blood and fluids. Alternatively, if the spleen is vacuous and fails to move and transform, water qì gathers, accumulates, and ascends to invade the heart. Both these conditions can result in water qì or water-rheum congealing and binding in the heart. These are pathomechanisms that are involved in water congealing in the blood vessels and water qì flooding and spilling.

水犯于心

血的主要成分是营气和津液。心主血脉，心气在推动血液运行的同时，也能推动津液运行。如果心气虚弱，不能行血，也不能运行津液，或者脾虚失运，水气停留，上犯于心，均可导致水气、水饮凝结于心，出现水凝血脉和水气泛溢的病机变化。

4.1 Water Congealing in the Blood Vessels

When water qì and water-rheum invade the heart, they impede the movement of qì and blood. This deprives the blood vessels of nourishment and unsettles the heart spirit, causing heart palpitations or fearful throbbing. When heart qì is impeded, the ancestral qì is weakened and the breathing becomes inhibited. This causes oppression in the chest and shortness of breath. When the heart vessels are impeded and channel qì lacks free flow, heart and chest pain result. When the qì in the vessels is unable to move with continuity, the pulse quality will be either bound or intermittent.

Water qì and water-rheum are pathological products that are invariably engendered by vacuity. Although a condition of root vacuity and tip repletion arises as soon as water qì is formed and water-rheum accumulates, the pathomechanism is governed by repletion. It should be treated by supplementing the heart and freeing the vessels while transforming qì and moving water. For a formula to treat this condition, use Woody Fangji Decoction (*mù fáng jǐ tāng*) from the *Jīn Guì Yào Lüè* ("Essential Prescriptions of the Golden Coffer"), with the addition of Chinese angelica, chuanxiong, and salvia.

Woody Fangji Decoction (木防己汤 *mù fáng jǐ tāng*)

fáng jǐ (防己 Stephaniae Tetrandrae Radix, fangji)
guì zhī (桂枝 Cinnamomi Ramulus, cinnamon twig)
huáng qí (黄芪 Astragali Radix, astragalus)
dǎng shēn (党参 Codonopsis Radix, codonopsis)
fú líng (茯苓 Poria, poria)
bái zhú (白术 Atractylodis Macrocephalae Rhizoma, white atractylodes)
Plus:
dāng guī (当归 Angelicae Sinensis Radix, Chinese angelica)
chuān xiōng (川芎 Chuanxiong Rhizoma, chuanxiong)
dān shēn (丹参 Salviae Miltiorrhizae Radix, salvia)

水凝血脉

水气、水饮犯心，阻碍气血的运行，心脉失养，心神不宁，则为心悸怔忡；阻碍心气，宗气因而衰少，呼吸不利，则胸闷短气；阻碍心脉，经气不通，则心胸疼痛；脉气不能续接，则脉象或结或代。水气、水饮是病理产物，必因虚而生，一旦形成水气、水饮停留，则产生本虚标实，以实为主的病机。治宜补心通脉，化气行水。方用《金匮要略》加减木防己汤（木防己、桂枝、黄芪、党参、茯苓、白术）加当归、川芎、丹参进行治疗。

Literature Review of Water Congealing in the Blood Vessels

📖 *Jīn Guì Yào Lüè* ("Essential Prescriptions of the Golden Coffer"), "Chapter on Phlegm-Rheum Cough"

"Whenever patients drink copious amounts of water, they invariably suffer from fulminant panting and fullness. In all cases of reduced intake of food and copious intake of fluids, water will collect below the heart. In severe cases, it will lead to palpitations. In mild cases, it will lead to shortness of breath."

This quotation points out that water qì and water-rheum intimidating the heart will impede the movement of qì and blood and deprive the heart vessels of nourishment. This can lead to pathoconditions that present with heart palpitations and shortness of breath.

《金匮要略•痰饮咳嗽篇》说："夫病人饮水多，必暴喘满。凡食少饮多，水停心下。甚者则悸，微者短气。"指出水气、水饮凌心，阻碍气血运行，心脉失养，可致心悸、气短等症。

4.2 Water Qì Flooding and Spilling

Water qì and water-rheum invade the heart if they are not coursed and dissipated. If water qì and water-rheum flood and spill into the interstices below the skin, the entire body will have mild puffy swelling. Water qì and water-rheum may also ascend counterflow to invade the clear orifices, influencing the ascent of clear yáng qì to nourish the head and eyes. This results in dizziness and blurred vision.

If water qì and water-rheum collect below the heart and obstruct stomach qì, there will be distention and fullness below the heart. If water qì is not transformed and is unable to descend to the bladder to form urine, it will result in short and scant urine. This should be treated by warming and freeing heart qì while transforming qì and moving water. For a formula, use Poria, Cinnamon Twig, White Atractylodes, and Licorice Decoction (*líng guì zhú gān tāng*) from the *Jīn Guì Yào Lüè* ("Essential Prescriptions of the Golden Coffer"), with the addition of alisma and coix.

Poria, Cinnamon Twig, White Atractylodes, and Licorice Decoction
(苓桂朮甘汤 *líng guì zhú gān tāng*)

---

fú líng (茯苓 Poria, poria)
guì zhī (桂枝 Cinnamomi Ramulus, cinnamon twig)
bái zhú (白朮 Atractylodis Macrocephalae Rhizoma, white atractylodes)
gān cǎo (甘草 Glycyrrhizae Radix, licorice)
Plus:
zé xiè (泽泻 Alismatis Rhizoma, alisma)
yì yǐ rén (薏苡仁 Coicis Semen, coix)

水气泛溢

水气、水饮犯心，不得疏散。水气、水饮泛溢于肌腠皮下，则引起全身轻度浮肿；水气、水饮上逆，上犯清窍，影响清阳之气上养头目，则为头目眩晕；水气、水饮停于心下，阻滞胃气，则为心下胀满；水气不化，不能下输膀胱生成尿液，则小便短少。治宜温通心气，化气行水。方用《金匮要略》苓桂术甘汤（茯苓、桂枝、白术、甘草）加泽泻、薏苡。

Literature Review of Water Qì Flooding and Spilling

📖 *Jīn Guì Yào Lüè* ("Essential Prescriptions of the Golden Coffer"), "Chapter on Phlegm-Rheum Cough"

"In cases of phlegm-rheum below the heart with propping fullness in the chest and rib-sides and blurred vision, Poria, Cinnamon Twig, White Atractylodes, and Licorice Decoction (*líng guì zhú gān tāng*) governs."

This quotation points out that water collecting below the heart impedes stomach qì and can lead to distention and fullness in the stomach, stomach duct, chest, and rib-sides. Clear yáng failing to ascend may cause dizziness.

文献评述

《金匮要略•痰饮咳嗽篇》说："心下有痰饮，胸胁支满，目眩，苓桂术甘汤主之。"指出水停心下，阻碍胃气，可致胃脘、胸胁胀满；清阳不升，可致头眩。"

Summary of Water Invading the Heart

1. Water Congealing in the Blood Vessels
   Vessel qì deprived of nourishment: Heart palpitations, fearful throbbing, oppression in the chest, and shortness of breath
   Vessel qì failing to move freely: Heart and chest pain
   Discontinuity of vessel qì: A pulse that is bound or intermittent
2. Water Qì Flooding and Spilling
   Water flooding the entire body: Generalized water swelling and inhibited urination
   Water qì flooding upwards: Dizziness
   Water collecting below the heart: Distention and fullness below the heart

---

水犯于心

水凝血脉
　　脉气失养 —— 心悸怔忡，胸闷气短。
　　脉气不通 —— 心胸疼痛。
　　脉气不续 —— 脉结或代。
水气泛溢
　　水泛全身 —— 全身水肿，小便不利。
　　水气上泛 —— 头晕目眩。
　　水停心下 —— 心下胀满。

Chapter Five

Blood Stasis in the Heart

Qì stagnation, qì vacuity, blood cold, and blood heat may all give rise to static blood. Static blood is not only a pathological product; it is also a new pathogenic factor. Static blood invading the heart viscus is the pathomechanism that causes static blood obstructing the vessels and static blood blocking the spirit.

血瘀于心

由于气滞、气虚、血寒、血热等各种原因可引起瘀血。瘀血既是病理产物，又是新的致病因素，侵犯心脏，导致瘀血阻脉和瘀血闭神的病机变化。

5.1 Static Blood Obstructing the Vessels

Damage from the seven affects causes emotional depression, qì stagnation from lack of free flow, and static movement of blood. Alternatively, taxation fatigue and enduring illness can damage the heart, causing insufficiency of heart qì, failure of the qì to move the blood, and blood stagnation in the vessels. All these factors can cause stasis and obstruction in the heart vessels.

When the heart vessels are obstructed, blood cannot nourish the heart. This causes heart stirring, which leads to heart palpitations, fearful throbbing, oppression in the chest, and shortness of breath. Static blood may obstruct the blood vessels in the body of the heart, as well as in the area of the hand lesser yīn heart channel. If the channel qì fails to flow freely, it manifests as stifling oppression and stabbing pain in the heart and chest that radiates into the chest and back, as well as pain in the medial and posterior edges of the hands and arms. The stasis obstructs the network vessels of the tongue body and the color of the static blood appears externally, manifesting in a darkened tongue color or stasis macules and stasis speckles.

This condition should be treated by quickening the blood and transforming stasis while regulating qì and freeing the network vessels. For conditions of qì stagnation and blood stasis, use the formula House of Blood Stasis-Expelling Decoction (*xuè fǔ zhú yū tāng*) from the text *Yī Lín Gǎi Cuò* ("Correction of Errors in Medical Classics").

House of Blood Stasis-Expelling Decoction
(血府逐瘀汤 *xuè fǔ zhú yū tāng*)

chái hú (柴胡 Bupleuri Radix, bupleurum)
bái sháo (白芍 Paeoniae Radix Alba, white peony)
dāng guī (当归 Angelicae Sinensis Radix, Chinese angelica)
chuān xiōng (川芎 Chuanxiong Rhizoma, chuanxiong)
shēng dì huáng (生地黄 Rehmanniae Radix Exsiccata seu Recens,
    dried/fresh rehmannia)
táo rén (桃仁 Persicae Semen, peach kernel)
hóng huā (红花 Carthami Flos, carthamus)
zhǐ qiào (ké) (枳壳 Aurantii Fructus, bitter orange)
niú xī (牛膝 Achyranthis Bidentatae Radix, achyranthes)
gān cǎo (甘草 Glycyrrhizae Radix, licorice)

For conditions of qì vacuity with blood stasis, use the formula Peach Kernel and Carthamus Four Agents Decoction (*táo hóng sì wù tāng*) from the *Yī Zōng Jīn Jiàn* ("The Golden Mirror of Orthodox Medicine"), with the addition of typha pollen, notoginseng, ginseng, cinnamon twig, and stinkbug.

Peach Kernel and Carthamus Four Agents Decoction
(桃红四物汤 *táo hóng sì wù tāng*)

táo rén (桃仁 Persicae Semen, peach kernel)
hóng huā (红花 Carthami Flos, carthamus)
chuān xiōng (川芎 Chuanxiong Rhizoma, chuanxiong)
dāng guī (当归 Angelicae Sinensis Radix, Chinese angelica)
chì sháo (赤芍 Paeoniae Radix Rubra, red peony)
shēng dì huáng (生地黄 Rehmanniae Radix Exsiccata seu Recens,
    dried/fresh rehmannia)
Plus:
pú huáng (蒲黄 Typhae Pollen, typha pollen)
sān qī (三七 Notoginseng Radix, notoginseng)
rén shēn (人参 Ginseng Radix, ginseng)
guì zhī (桂枝 Cinnamomi Ramulus, cinnamon twig)
jiǔ xiāng chóng (九香虫 Aspongopus, stinkbug)

瘀血阻脉

七情所伤，情志郁结，气滞不通，血行瘀滞；或劳倦、久病伤心，心气不足，气不行血，血滞脉中，均可瘀阻心脉。心脉阻滞，血不养心，心动不宁，则为心悸怔忡，胸闷气短；瘀血阻滞心体血脉和手少阴心经经脉循行部位，经气不通，则为心胸憋闷刺痛，牵引胸背、手臂内侧后缘疼痛。阻滞舌体络脉，瘀血之色外现，则为舌色晦暗，或有瘀斑、瘀点。

治宜活血化瘀，理气通络。以气滞血瘀为主者，可用《医林改错》血府逐瘀汤（柴胡、白芍、当归、川芎、生地、桃仁、红花、枳壳、牛膝、甘草）；以气虚血瘀为主者，方用《医宗金鉴》桃红四物汤（桃仁、红花、川芎、当归、赤芍、生地）加蒲黄、三七、人参、桂枝、九香虫。

5.2 Static Blood Blocking the Spirit

Heat entering the blood chamber in women and heat binding in the bladder cause poor qì transformation. Stasis and heat bind with each other and may ascend to harass the heart spirit, causing manic derangement of the heart spirit and disquietude. The manic mental derangement occurs regardless of who is present. The nature of static blood is yīn; thus, at night when yīn qì is more exuberant, the severity of blood stasis increases. This makes the mental derangement more severe at night.

The liver stores the blood and opens into the orifices of the eyes. If static blood impedes the nourishment of blood to the upper body, it may cause blurred vision. The patient will develop flowery vision and confusion; the symptoms are as if they are seeing ghosts.

Stasis and heat binding together and harassing the heart spirit should be treated by clearing heat and draining fire while quickening the blood and transforming stasis. For a formula, use Peach Kernel Qì-Infusing Decoction (*táo hé chéng qì tāng*) from *Shāng Hán Lùn* ("On Cold Damage"), with the addition of salvia and red peony.

Peach Kernel Qì-Infusing Decoction (桃核承气汤 *táo hé chéng qì tāng*)
táo rén (桃仁 Persicae Semen, peach kernel)
dāng guī (当归 Angelicae Sinensis Radix, Chinese angelica)
bái sháo (白芍 Paeoniae Radix Alba, white peony)
mǔ dān pí (牡丹皮 Moutan Cortex, moutan)
dà huáng (大黄 Rhei Radix et Rhizoma, rhubarb)
máng xiāo (芒硝 Natrii Sulfas, mirabilite)
Plus:
dān shēn (丹参 Salviae Miltiorrhizae Radix, salvia)
chì sháo (赤芍 Paeoniae Radix Rubra, red peony)

瘀血闭神

妇人热入血室，或热结膀胱，气化不行，瘀热互结，上扰心神，心神狂乱，不得安宁，故精神狂乱，不避亲疏；瘀血性质属阴，到了夜晚，阴气偏盛，加重血瘀的程度，故入夜神志错乱加重；肝藏血，开窍于目，瘀血阻碍，血不上养，视力模糊，故病人感到眼花缭乱，如见鬼状。

由于是瘀热互结，扰乱心神，故治宜清热泻火，活血化瘀。方用《伤寒论》桃核承气汤（桃仁、当归、芍药、牡丹皮、大黄、芒硝）加丹参、赤芍。

Literature Review of Blood Stasis in the Heart

📖 *Shāng Hán Lùn* ("On Cold Damage"), "Sixth Entry on Pulse, Pattern Identification, and Treatment of Greater Yáng Disease"

> "When greater yáng disease is not resolved, heat binds in the bladder and the patient acts as if manic. If there is a tense bound lesser abdomen after external resolution, attacking may be used; Peach Kernel Qì-Infusing Decoction (*táo hé chéng qì tāng*) is appropriate."

This points out that if heat binds in the bladder, brewing of heat evils can concentrate the blood and produce stasis. Stasis and heat binding together can ascend to harass the heart spirit, resulting in manic derangement of the essence-spirit.

📖 *Shāng Hán Lùn* ("On Cold Damage"), "Seventh Entry on Pulse, Pattern Identification, and Treatment of Greater Yáng Disease"

> "When there is cold damage in women [that presents with] heat effusion, timely menstruation, and clarity during the day and delirious speech after dusk, with symptoms as if they were seeing ghosts, this is a case of heat entering the blood chamber."

This quote points out that when heat enters the blood chamber and binds with blood, it can cause stasis heat to harass the upper body, resulting in manic derangement of the essence-spirit.

文献评述

《伤寒论·辨太阳病脉证并治第六》说："太阳病不解，热结膀胱，其人如狂，……外解已，少腹急结者，乃可攻之，宜桃核承气汤。"指出热结膀胱，热邪煎熬，血液浓缩瘀滞，瘀热互结，上扰心神，可致精神狂乱。

《伤寒论·辨太阳病脉证并治第七》说："妇人伤寒，发热，经水适来，昼日明了，暮则谵语，如见鬼状者，此为热入血室。"指出热入血室，热与血结，瘀热上扰，可致精神狂乱。

Summary of Blood Stasis in the Heart

1. Static Blood Obstructing the Vessels
 	
    Heart vessels deprived of nourishment: Heart palpitations, fearful throbbing, oppression in the chest, and shortness of breath
    Heart vessel obstruction: Stifling oppression and stabbing pain in the heart and chest that stretches through the chest, back, and the inside of the arms
    Stasis obstructing the network vessels of the tongue: Darkened tongue color, sometimes with stasis macules or stasis speckles
2. Static Blood Blocking the Spirit
    Ascending to harass the heart spirit: Manic mental derangement regardless of who is present that is exacerbated in the evening
    Ascending to harass the eyes: Flowery vision and symptoms of confusion as if seeing ghosts

血瘀于心

瘀血阻脉
    心脉失养 —— 心悸怔忡，胸闷气短。
    心脉痹阻 —— 心胸憋闷刺痛，牵引胸背、臂内疼痛。
    舌络瘀阻 —— 舌色晦暗，或有瘀斑、瘀点。
瘀血闭神
    上扰心神 —— 精神狂乱，不避亲疏，入夜尤甚。
    上扰于目 —— 眼花缭乱，如见鬼状。

Chapter Six

Heart Repletion Cold

The heart may be influenced by both externally contracted cold evil assailing the outer body and by internally engendered cold rheum invading the inner body. The pathomechanisms involved in heart repletion cold are explained as the violent struggle between evil and right. Heart repletion cold is caused by either disease evils or by the presence of pathological products. Because of the difference in pathological causes, the pathomechanisms of heart repletion cold can be divided into two main categories: cold evil damaging the heart and cold rheum invading the heart.

心实寒

外感寒邪，或内生寒饮，外袭内犯，均可影响于心。由于有病邪或病理产物的存在，邪正斗争激烈，从而形成心实寒的病机。根据致病原因的差异，心实寒的病机可分为寒邪伤心和寒饮犯心两大类。

6.1 Cold Evil Damaging the Heart

Externally contracted cold evils may strike directly into the interior to invade the heart. Cold governs contraction and tautness and is congealing and stagnating. Cold evils invading the inner body cause congealing in the heart vessels and stagnation of the heart qì. This process is involved in the pathomechanisms of cold damaging heart yáng, cold congealing in the heart vessels, and cold blocking the heart spirit.

寒邪伤心

外感寒邪，直中于里，可内犯于心。寒主收引、凝滞，寒邪内犯，凝滞心气心脉，可引起寒伤心阳、寒凝心脉和寒闭心神的病机变化。

6.1.1   Cold Damaging Heart Yáng

Yáng qì governs the entire body. The heart holds the office of monarch, but it is only able to perform its functions as a monarch when it receives nourishment from yáng qì. Cold is a yīn evil that enters from the outside and can easily damage the yáng qì of the heart, causing it to be useless as a monarch. When cold evil invades the heart, the destructive power of yīn cold blocks the qì dynamic. This results in cold pain within the heart, chest, and back that worsens upon contraction of cold but is relieved by heat.

Cold damaging heart yáng causes a loss of warmth. As a result, qì and blood cannot ascend to provide luxuriance to the face; thus, the blood vessels in the face lose fullness. This leads to a somber white facial complexion and a pale tongue with white fur. When yáng qì is unable to warm the entire body and the four limbs, there is aversion to cold, a curled-up lying posture, and reversal cold in the extremities. This condition arises from the contraction of cold and is ascribed to the pathomechanism of heart repletion; this is because heart yáng has been damaged but it has not reached the point of vacuity detriment. The suitable treatment is to dispel and dissipate cold evil while warming and freeing heart yáng. For a formula, choose Cinnamon Twig Decoction (*guì zhī tāng*) from *Shāng Hán Lùn* ("On Cold Damage"), with the addition of aconite, ginseng, notopterygium, saposhnikovia, and turmeric.

Cinnamon Twig Decoction (桂枝汤 *guì zhī tāng*)
guì zhī (桂枝 Cinnamomi Ramulus, cinnamon twig)
bái sháo (白芍 Paeoniae Radix Alba, white peony)
shēng jiāng (生姜 Zingiberis Rhizoma Recens, fresh ginger)
dà zǎo (大枣 Jujubae Fructus, jujube)
gān cǎo (甘草 Glycyrrhizae Radix, licorice)
Plus:
fù zǐ (附子 Aconiti Radix Lateralis Praeparata, aconite)
rén shēn (人参 Ginseng Radix, ginseng)
qiāng huó (羌活 Notopterygii Rhizoma et Radix, notopterygium)
fáng fēng (防风 Saposhnikoviae Radix, saposhnikovia)
jiāng huáng (姜黄 Curcumae Longae Rhizoma, turmeric)

寒伤心阳

人之一身，阳气为主。心为君主之官，得阳气濡养，方能行使君主之事。寒为阴邪，自外而入，易伤心的阳气，而失君主之用。寒邪犯心，阴寒肃杀，气机闭塞，则心中胸背冷痛，受寒加重，得热则缓；寒伤心阳，不能温煦气血上荣于面，面部血脉失充，则面色苍白，舌淡苔白；阳气不能温煦全身、四肢，则恶寒蜷卧、手足厥冷。此因受寒而起，心阳虽受伤害，但未致虚损，故仍属心实的病机。治宜祛散寒邪，温通心阳。方选《伤寒论》<u>桂枝汤</u>（桂枝、芍药、生姜、大枣、甘草）加附子、人参、羌活、防风、姜黄。

6.1.2 Cold Congealing in the Heart Vessels

In cases of external contraction of cold evil, heart qì fails to spread and propel the movement of blood. This is because cold governs contraction and tautness, and it congeals and retracts heart qì. Congealing and stagnation from cold cause the blood to lose its warmth and free flow, resulting in cold blood that moves slowly. These factors can produce obstruction in the heart vessels, giving rise to pathoconditions that present with congestion of qì in the chest, shortness of breath, and cold pain in the heart and chest.

In cases of either sudden fulminant contraction of cold evil or cases of constitutional yáng vacuity with contraction of cold evil, yīn overwhelms the position of yáng, causing heart qì to suddenly retract. This results in cold congealing the heart vessels, which leads to severe blood stasis. The resulting pathocondition manifests with sudden chest pain, severe pain, cold pain, either heart pain stretching through to the back or back pain stretching through to the heart, cough and spitting that induces pain, blue-green cold extremities, and a somber facial complexion.

True heart pain can result from periods of severe congealing cold. As stated in the *Líng Shū* ("The Magic Pivot"), "On Reversal," this pathocondition manifests externally as "blue-green coloration in the extremities extending to the joints, along with severe heart pain, and a morning onset with death in the evening or an evening onset with death in the morning." A suitable treatment is warming and dissipating cold evil while quickening the blood and transforming stasis. For treatment, use the formula Aconite Main Tuber and Halloysite Pill (*wū tóu chì shí zhī wán*) from the *Jīn Guì Yào Lüè* ("Essential Prescriptions of the Golden Coffer"), with the addition of ligusticum, salvia, and red peony.

Aconite Main Tuber and Halloysite Pill (乌头赤石脂丸 *wū tóu chì shí zhī wán*)
wū tóu, aconite (乌头 Aconiti Radix Wutou) *chì shí zhī* (赤石脂 Halloysitum Rubrum, halloysite) *fù zǐ* (附子 Aconiti Radix Lateralis Praeparata, aconite) *gān jiāng* (干姜 Zingiberis Rhizoma, dried ginger)

huā jiāo (花椒 Zanthoxyli Pericarpium, zanthoxylum)

Plus:

chuān xiōng (川芎 Chuanxiong Rhizoma, chuanxiong)
dān shēn (丹参 Salviae Miltiorrhizae Radix, salvia)
chì sháo (赤芍 Paeoniae Radix Rubra, red peony)

寒凝心脉

外感寒邪，寒主收引，凝缩心气，心气不展，不能推动血行；寒主凝滞，不能温通血液，血寒运行迟慢，均可导致心脉痹阻，引起胸中气塞、短气、心胸冷痛等症。

若卒然暴感寒邪，或素体阳虚,复感寒邪，阴乘阳位，心气暴缩，心脉寒凝，血瘀严重则见胸痛暴作、剧痛、冷痛，心痛彻背,背痛彻心，咳唾引痛，手足青冷面色晦暗等症。

寒凝严重时则为真心痛，外见"手足青至节，心痛甚，旦发夕死，夕发旦死"等症（《灵枢•厥论》）。治宜温散寒邪，活血化瘀。方用《金匮要略》乌头赤石脂丸（乌头、赤石脂、附子、干姜、蜀椒）加川芎、丹参、赤芍进行治疗。

Literature Review of Cold Congealing in the Heart Vessels

📖 *Sù Wèn* ("Plain Questions"), "Treatise on Regulating the Channels"

> "If cold qì accumulates in the chest and is not drained, warm qì departs and cold alone remains, resulting in congealed blood. Congealing causes a lack of free flow in the vessels."

This quotation points out that cold congealing in the blood vessels can lead to obstruction of the heart vessels.

📖 *Zhū Bìng Yuán Hòu Lùn* ("The Origin and Indicators of Disease"), "Symptoms of Painful Heart Disorders"

> "Heart pain is caused by wind-cold evil qì overwhelming the heart."

This quotation points out that cold evil can congeal in the heart vessels and give rise to heart pain.

📖 *Jīn Guì Yào Lüè* ("Essential Prescriptions of the Golden Coffer"), "Chapter on Wind-Cold Accumulations and Gatherings in the Five Viscera"

> "In cases of cold inside the heart, the patient will suffer from disorders of the heart, as if in a state of overeating garlic. In severe cases, heart pain will stretch to the back or back pain will stretch to the chest, resembling an influx of *gǔ*."

This quotation points out that a direct strike of external cold can cause congealing in the heart vessels and pain stretching through the chest and back.

📖 *Shèng Jì Zŏng Lù* ("Sages' Salvation Records"), "Chest Impediment and Chest Pain"

"Chest pain belongs to the category of chest impediment. It is caused by general vacuity complicated by wind and is exacerbated by cold qì. It manifests as stabbing pain in the anterior chest and the region of the breasts. In severe cases, the pain stretches into the back and shoulder blades or stretches to the back and spine, with coughing and spitting that induce pain."

This quotation explains that pain stretching through the chest and back can result from contraction of cold evil by a person with general vacuity as well as from cold congealing in the heart vessels.

文献评述

《素问•调经论》说："寒气积于胸中而不泻，不泻则温气去，寒独留则血凝泣，凝则脉不通。"指出寒凝血脉，可致心脉痹阻。

《诸病源候论•心痛病诸候》说："心痛者，风冷邪气乘于心也。"指出寒邪可凝滞心脉而引起心痛。

《金匮要略•五脏风寒积聚篇》说："心中寒者，其人苦病心如噉蒜状，剧者心痛彻背，背痛彻胸，譬如蛊注。"指出外寒直中，可引起心脉凝滞，胸背彻痛。

《圣济总录•胸痹•胸痛》说："胸痛者，胸痹之类也。此由体虚挟风，又遇寒气加之，则胸膺两乳间刺痛，甚则引背胛，或彻背膂，咳唾引痛是也。"解释了体虚之人受到寒邪侵袭，也会因寒凝心脉而致胸背彻痛。

6.1.3 Cold Blocking the Heart Spirit

When cold evil is contracted and it erupts right after striking, the cold evil very quickly directly strikes the three yīn, causing heart qì to congeal, which depresses and blocks the heart spirit. The heart spirit will be ungoverned, which can cause sudden collapse and clouding loss of consciousness. Cold governs contraction and tautness, and can cause patterns that present with a clenched jaw preventing speech, rigidity of the limbs, and hypertonicity and pain. The suitable treatment involves dissipating cold, opening the orifices, and arousing the spirit. For a formula, use Storax Pill (*sū hé xiāng wán*) from the *Tài Píng Huì Mín Hé Jì Jú Fāng* ("Tài-Píng Imperial Grace Pharmacy Formulas").

Storax Pill (苏合香丸 *sū hé xiāng wán*)

sū hé xiāng (苏合香 Styrax, storax)

rǔ xiāng (乳香 Olibanum, frankincense)

shè xiāng (麝香 Moschus, musk)

dīng xiāng (丁香 Caryophylli Flos, clove)

chén xiāng (沉香 Aquilariae Lignum Resinatum, aquilaria)

ān xī xiāng (安息香 Benzoinum, benzoin)

tán xiāng (檀香 Santali Albi Lignum, sandalwood)

mù xiāng (木香 Aucklandiae Radix, costusroot)

[chǎo] xiāng fù ([炒]香附 Cyperi Rhizoma, cyperus [stir-fried])

bái zhú (白朮 Atractylodis Macrocephalae Rhizoma, white atractylodes)

bì bō (荜茇 Piperis Longi Fructus, long pepper)

hē zǐ (诃子 Chebulae Fructus, chebule)

zhū shā (朱砂 Cinnabaris, cinnabar)

xī jiǎo (犀角 Rhinocerotis Cornu, rhinoceros horn)

bīng piàn (冰片 Borneolum, borneol)

寒闭心神

感受寒邪，随中随发，仓卒之间，寒邪直中三阴，凝滞心气，郁闭心神，心神无主，可致卒然倒仆、昏不知人；寒主收引，可致口噤不语、四肢强直、拘急疼痛等症。治宜散寒开窍醒神。方用《太平惠民和剂局方》苏合香丸。

Literature Review of Cold Blocking the Heart Spirit

📖 *Sù Wèn* ("Plain Questions"), "Treatise on Pain"

"When cold evil settles in the five viscera, it will cause reverse flow with discharge above and an exhaustion of yīn qì. Yáng qì cannot enter, causing sudden pain, death or loss of consciousness. When qì is restored, the person will live."

This quotation points out that cold settling in the five viscera mainly invades the heart, obstructing heart qì and causing chaotic counterflow of the qì dynamic. The heart spirit becomes harassed, which gives rise to clouding loss of consciousness.

📖 *Zá Bìng Yuán Liú Xī Zhú* ("Incisive Light on the Source of Miscellaneous Disease"), "The Source of Cold Disease"

"Cold strike refers to a direct strike of the three yīn by cold evil. It results in sudden clouding loss of consciousness, a clenched jaw, and rigidity, hypertonicity, and pain of the limbs."

This quotation points out that cold evil can directly invade the heart, obstructing heart qì and clouding the heart spirit. This gives rise to pathologies such as a clouded and fretting heart spirit and contraction and tautness of the limbs.

文献评述

《素问·举痛论》说："寒邪客于五脏，厥逆上泄，阴气竭，阳气未入，故卒然痛死不知人，气复返，则生矣。"指出寒客五脏，主要犯心，心气受阻，气机逆乱，心神受扰，从而引起昏不知人。

《杂病源流犀烛·寒病源流》说："中寒者，寒邪直中三阴，卒然昏不省人，口噤，四肢强直，拘急疼痛。"指出寒邪可直接犯心，痹阻心气，蒙蔽心神，引起心神昏愦、肢体收引的病变。

Summary of Cold Evil Damaging the Heart

1. Cold Damaging Heart Yáng
   Devitalized heart yáng: Cold pain in the heart, chest, and back that is exacerbated by cold and relieved by heat
   Loss of warmth in the face: Somber white facial complexion, pale tongue with white fur
   Loss of warmth in the trunk and limbs: Aversion to cold, lying in a curled-up posture, reversal cold of the extremities
2. Cold Congealing in the Heart Vessels
   Mild patterns: Congestion of qì in the chest, shortness of breath, cold pain in the heart and chest
   Severe patterns: Sudden chest pain, severe pain, cold pain, heart pain stretching into the back or back pain stretching into the heart, cough and spitting that induces pain, blue-green cold extremities, somber facial complexion
3. Cold Blocking the Heart Spirit
   Sudden collapse, clouding loss of consciousness, clenched jaw preventing speech, rigidity, hypertonicity, and pain of the limbs

寒邪伤心

寒伤心阳
　心阳不振 —— 心中胸背冷痛，受寒加重，得热则缓。
　面部失温 —— 面色苍白，舌淡苔白。
　身肢失温 —— 恶寒蜷卧、手足厥冷。

寒凝心脉
　　轻证——胸中气塞、短气、心胸冷痛。
　　重证——胸痛暴作、剧痛、冷痛，心痛彻背，背痛彻心，咳唾
　　引痛，手足青冷，面色晦暗。
寒闭心神
　　卒然倒仆、昏不知人、口噤不语、四肢强直、拘急疼痛

6.2 Cold Rheum Invading the Heart

Cold rheum invading the heart refers to the pathomechanism by which cold phlegm or water-rheum collecting below the heart ascends to invade the heart. Normally, it is preceded by spleen-kidney yáng vacuity with forceless movement and qì transformation failure, which results in poor distribution of water and liquids. Cold phlegm or water-rheum are formed and collect below the heart, impeding the qì dynamic and giving rise to a feeling of glomus and fullness below the heart.

If the cold rheum below the heart proceeds further and ascends counterflow to obstruct the heart vessels, it will stretch into the heart and chest, resulting in heart and chest pain. If cold rheum invades the lungs and causes obstruction of lung qì, the result is oppression, distention, and fullness in the chest; coughing and vomiting with large amounts of white clear thin sputum may also result. This condition is associated with the pathomechanism of heart repletion cold because of the presence of large amounts of cold phlegm and water-rheum. Even though it originally stems from vacuity, it is considered to be a repletion condition because of the accumulation of pathological products. It should be treated by freeing yáng and dissipating cold while warming and transforming water-rheum. To treat this condition, use the formula Cinnamon Twig, Fresh Ginger, and Unripe Bitter Orange Decoction (*guì zhī shēng jiāng zhǐ shí tāng*) from the *Jīn Guì Yào Lüè* ("Essential Prescriptions of the Golden Coffer"), with the addition of raw arisaema, asarum, pinellia, poria, and tangerine peel.

> ### Cinnamon Twig, Fresh Ginger, and Unripe Bitter Orange Decoction
> ### (桂枝生姜枳实汤 *guì zhī shēng jiāng zhǐ shí tāng*)
>
> *guì zhī* (桂枝 Cinnamomi Ramulus, cinnamon twig)
> *shēng jiāng* (生姜 Zingiberis Rhizoma Recens, fresh ginger)
> *zhǐ shí* (枳实 Aurantii Fructus Immaturus, unripe bitter orange)
> Plus:
> *shēng nán xīng* (生南星 Arisaematis Rhizoma Crudum, unprocessed arisaema)

xì xīn (细辛 Asari Herba, asarum)
bàn xià (半夏 Pinelliae Rhizoma, pinellia)
fú líng (茯苓 Poria, poria)
chén pí (陈皮 Citri Reticulatae Pericarpium, tangerine peel)

寒饮犯心

寒饮犯心是指寒痰或水饮停于心下，上犯于心而引起的病机变化。一般先有脾肾阳虚，推动乏力，气化不行，水津失布，形成寒痰水饮，停聚心下，阻碍气机，引起心下痞满之感。心下寒饮进一步上逆，痹阻心脉，则牵引心胸，引起心胸疼痛；寒饮上犯于肺，肺气阻滞，则为胸闷胀满，咳嗽呕吐大量色白清稀痰液。由于有大量寒痰水饮存在，虽然因虚而致，但有病理产物停留，仍为心实寒的病机所致。治宜通阳散寒，温化水饮。方用《金匮要略》桂枝生姜枳实汤（桂枝、生姜、枳实）加生南星、细辛、半夏、茯苓、陈皮进行调治。

Literature Review of Cold Rheum Invading the Heart

📖 *Jīn Guì Yào Lüè* ("Essential Prescriptions of the Golden Coffer"), "Ninth Entry on Pulse, Pattern Identification and Treatment of Chest Impediment, Heart Pain, and Shortness of Breath"

"For glomus in the heart and all counterflow with suspended pain in the heart, Cinnamon Twig, Fresh Ginger, and Unripe Bitter Orange Decoction (*guì zhī shēng jiāng zhǐ shí tāng*) governs."

This quote points out that phlegm-rheum collecting below the heart that ascends to invade the heart can cause obstruction of the heart vessels, resulting in heart pain.

文献评述

《金匮要略•胸痹心痛短气病脉证治第九》说："心中痞，诸逆心悬痛，桂枝生姜枳实汤主之。"指出痰饮停于心下，上犯于心，痹阻心脉，可引起心痛。

Summary of Cold Rheum Invading the Heart

1. Obstruction of Stomach Qì
   Glomus and fullness below the heart

2. Obstruction of the Heart Vessels

   Heart and chest pain
3. Obstruction of Lung Qì

   Oppression, distention, and fullness in the chest, cough and vomiting
   with large amounts of white clear thin sputum

寒饮犯心

阻滞胃气
    心下痞满。
痹阻心脉
    心胸疼痛。
阻滞肺气
    胸闷胀满，咳嗽呕吐大量色白清稀痰液。

Chapter Seven

Heart Repletion Heat

Many pathomechanisms lead to heart repletion heat. Fire from external or internal causes may invade the heart to produce heart repletion heat. Externally contracted evil qì may transform into fire from the conditions of wind-heat, dryness-heat, damp-heat, or cold-damp. Fire may also result from internal causes such as internally engendered phlegm fire, or fire formation from emotional depression. Harm results from hyperactivity due to exuberant heart yáng, and qì in superabundance becomes fire. Because all these conditions produce fire that can invade the heart, they are all involved in the pathomechanisms of heart repletion heat. These pathomechanisms can be divided into several categories: evil heat harassing the spirit, phlegm fire harassing the heart, heat hurrying the blood in the vessels, and fire flaming upward or spreading downward.

心实热

外感风热、燥热、湿热邪气，或寒湿之邪化火，或内生痰火，或情志郁结化火，或心的阳气亢盛，亢则为害，气有余则是火，均可犯及于心，引起心的实热病机。其病机变化可分为邪热扰神，痰火扰心、热迫血脉、上炎下移等几个方面。

7.1 Evil Heat Harassing the Spirit

The heart governs the spirit-mind. The activity of the heart spirit is smooth, regulated, and harmonious when there is tranquility, but harassment by evil qì is difficult for the heart to bear. The heart is a yáng viscus ascribed to fire according to the five phases, so it is particularly susceptible to the evil qì of wind, summerheat, heat, and fire. In addition to these factors, emotional depression and qì depression transforming into fire can easily give rise to hyperactivity of heart yáng. When the heart spirit is harassed and stirred, it gives rise to various symptoms of the spirit-mind associated with agitation. The pathomechanisms of this disorder can be divided into the manifestations of heart fire harassing the spirit, heat falling into the pericardium, or heat entering the heart construction.

邪热扰神

心主神志，心神活动以和为调，宁静为顺，难于忍受邪气干扰。心为阳脏，五行属火，对风、暑、热、火等邪气有着特殊的易感性。或因情志郁结，气郁化火，均易引起心阳易亢，扰动心神，引起躁扰不安等各种神志症状。其病机表现可分为心火扰神，热陷心包，热入心营等几个方面。

7.1.1 Heart Fire Harassing the Spirit

An exuberance of heart fire has a variety of causes. It may result from binding depression of the seven affects, fire formation due to excess among the five minds, or excessive exuberance of visceral qì. Exuberant heart fire may also result from over-consumption of acrid, spicy, hot, and drying foods or excessive ingestion of acrid and dry medicinals. In repletion heart fire, the heat resides in the qì aspect. Interior heat is rampant when there is effulgent fire in the heart. Internal heat brews and steams to harass the heart spirit. This causes heart yáng to float and stir, and the spirit will fail to keep to its abode. This will result in various symptoms of agitation.

In mild cases of harassment where the heart spirit only experiences slight harassment and stirring, the harassment merely results in a disquieted heart spirit and does not cause derangement. This manifests in heart palpitations and heart vexation, heat and oppression in the chest, anguish, tossing and turning, insomnia, and excessive dreaming. It should be treated by clearing heat and eliminating vexation while quieting the heart and spirit. For a formula, use Gardenia and Fermented Soybean Decoction (*zhī zǐ chǐ tāng*) from the *Shāng Hán Lùn* ("On Cold Damage"), together with Cinnabar Spirit-Quieting Pill (*zhū shā ān shén wán*) from the *Lán Shì Mì Cáng* ("Secret Treasure of the Orchid Chamber").

Gardenia and Fermented Soybean Decoction (栀子豉汤 *zhī zǐ chǐ tāng*)
zhī zǐ (栀子 Gardeniae Fructus, gardenia)
dàn dòu chǐ (淡豆豉 Sojae Semen Praeparatum, fermented soybean)

Cinnabar Spirit-Quieting Pill (朱砂安神丸 *zhū shā ān shén wán*)
huáng lián (黄连 Coptidis Rhizoma, coptis)
zhū shā (朱砂 Cinnabaris, cinnabar)
shēng dì huáng (生地黄 Rehmanniae Radix Exsiccata seu Recens, dried/fresh rehmannia)
dāng guī (当归 Angelicae Sinensis Radix, Chinese angelica)
zhì gān cǎo (炙甘草 Glycyrrhizae Radix cum Liquido Fricta, mix-fried licorice)

In serious cases, the heart spirit suffers from severe harassment. This produces agitation and stirring of the heart spirit and causes derangement and loss of memory. It will manifest in symptoms of clouded spirit, delirious speech, and incessant laughing. This should be treated by draining fire and clearing heat while settling the heart and quieting the spirit. For a formula, choose Heart-Draining Decoction (*xiè xīn tāng*) from the *Jīn Guì Yào Lüè* ("Essential Prescriptions of the Golden Coffer"), together with Iron Flakes Beverage (*shēng tiě luò yǐn*) from the text *Yī Xué Xīn Wù* ("Medical Insights").

Heart-Draining Decoction (泻心汤 *xiè xīn tāng*)
dà huáng (大黄 Rhei Radix et Rhizoma, rhubarb)
huáng lián (黄连 Coptidis Rhizoma, coptis)
huáng qín (黄芩 Scutellariae Radix, scutellaria)

Iron Flakes Beverage (生铁落饮 *shēng tiě luò yǐn*)
tiě luò (铁落 Ferri Frusta, iron flakes)
zhū shā (朱砂 Cinnabaris, cinnabar)
fú shén (茯神 Poria cum Pini Radice, root poria)
fú líng (茯苓 Poria, poria)
gōu téng (钩藤 Uncariae Ramulus cum Uncis, uncaria)
shí chāng pú (石菖蒲 Acori Tatarinowii Rhizoma, acorus)
dān shēn (丹参 Salviae Miltiorrhizae Radix, salvia)
lián qiào (连翘 Forsythiae Fructus, forsythia)
bèi mǔ (贝母 Fritillariae Bulbus, fritillaria)
dǎn xīng (胆星 Arisaema cum Bile, bile arisaema)
yuǎn zhì (远志 Polygalae Radix, polygala)
jú hóng (橘红 Citri Reticulatae Pericarpium Rubrum, red tangerine peel)
xuán shēn (玄参 Scrophulariae Radix, scrophularia)
tiān dōng (天冬 Asparagi Radix, asparagus)
mài dōng (麦冬 Ophiopogonis Radix, ophiopogon)

心火扰神

七情郁结，五志化火，或脏气过度亢盛，或过食辛辣燥热食物，或过服辛燥药品，均可致心火亢盛。此乃心之实火，热在气分。心中火旺，里热充斥，内热蕴蒸，心神被扰，心阳浮动，神不守舍，引起躁扰不安诸症。轻扰者，心神受到轻微扰动，仅为心神不宁，未至错乱，表现为心悸心烦，胸中热闷，懊憹颠倒，失眠多梦。治宜清热除烦，宁心安神。方选《伤寒论》栀子豉汤（栀子、豆豉）合《兰室秘藏》朱砂安神丸（黄连、朱砂、生地黄、当归、炙甘草）；重扰则心神受到严重干扰，心神躁动，错乱失志，可见神昏谵语，或喜笑不休等症。治宜泻火清热，镇心安神。方选《金匮要略》泻心汤（大黄、黄连、黄芩）合《医学心悟》生铁落饮（生铁落、朱砂、茯神、茯苓、钩藤、石菖蒲、丹参、连翘、贝母、胆星、远志、橘红、玄参、天冬、麦冬）。

Literature Review of Heart Fire Harassing the Spirit

📖 *Shèng Jì Zǒng Lù* ("Sages' Salvation Records"), "Vexing Heat in the Heart"

"Generally speaking, the heart is ascribed to fire and is averse to heat. It easily generates heat when it contracts disease; heat causes congestion of blood and qì. This results in vexation, agitation, and unquiet sleep."

This quotation points out that all cases of fire evil harassing and stirring the heart spirit can result in a disquieted heart spirit, manifesting with heart vexation and insomnia.

📖 *Sù Wèn* ("Plain Questions"), "Category of Fire"

"Agitation, stirring, vexation heat, harassment and disquietude are manifestations of fire. Severe heat in the outer body results in vexation and agitation of the limbs. Severe heat in the inner body results in agitation and stirring of the spirit-mind."

This quotation points out that when heart fire harasses the heart spirit internally, the spirit-mind will be disquieted, resulting in agitation.

📖 *Zhū Bìng Yuán Hòu Lùn* ("The Origin and Indicators of Disease"), "All Symptoms of Heart Disease"

"The heart and small intestine are linked in an interior-exterior relationship and both belong to the phase of fire, which is yáng qì. The heart governs the viscera, so its regular channel may not contract evil. If it is damaged by evil, there is pain and immediate death. If the branch and diverging network vessels are overwhelmed by wind evil there will be pain; if the condition endures, papules will occur. Pain, suspension, tension, and anguish are caused by evils hurrying yáng qì and inhibiting diffusion. This leads to congestion and stasis engendering heat; therefore, the heart is suspended and tense, with vexation, anguish, and pain."

This quotation points out that fire harassing the heart causes suspension and tension in the heart, possibly resulting in heart vexation and anguish.

📖 *Xuè Zhèng Lùn* ("Treatise on Blood Patterns"), "On Pathomechanisms of the Bowels and Viscera"

"When fire harasses the blood, it will cause anguish and a lack of brightness and clarity of the spirit. It leads to vacuity vexation, insomnia, stirring palpitations, fright, and fear."

The heart governs the blood and vessels. If fire harasses the blood, it will harass and stir the heart spirit. The result is a disquieted heart spirit, which gives rise to symptoms such as heart vexation and anguish, insomnia, and fright palpitations.

📖 *Zhū Bìng Yuán Hòu Lùn* ("The Origin and Indicators of Disease"), "Symptoms of Heart Disease"

> "Exuberance of heart qì refers to a superabundance of spirit…A tendency to laugh incessantly is a sign of heart qì repletion."

Qì in superabundance becomes fire. When heart qì is exuberant, it results in exuberant heart fire. This harasses the heart spirit and causes mental derangement, which gives rise to the tendency to laugh incessantly.

📖 *Jì Shēng Fāng* ("Formulas for Saving Lives"), "On Heart and Small Intestine Vacuity and Repletion"

> "As for their repletion, repletion engenders heat. Heat will cause vexation and derangement of the heart spirit, a red face and a hot body… susceptibility to laughing, fear, palpitations, and a pulse that is surging and replete. All these are symptoms of repletion heat."

This quotation points out that heat harassing the heart spirit causes heart vexation. In severe cases, it can cause mental derangement and incessant laughing.

📖 *Bǐ Huā Yī Jìng* ("*Bǐ Huā* Medical Mirror"), "Heart Section"

> "Heat in the heart refers to distress from fire, which causes vexation and agitation, sleeplessness, mania and withdrawal, and delirious speech."

This quotation points out that when repletion heat harasses the spirit, it causes hyperactivity and counterflow of heart yáng. The result is mental derangement, which is present in various pathomechanisms that affect the essence-spirit and are associated with mania.

文献评述

《圣济总录•心烦热》说："大抵心属火而恶热，其受病则易以生热，热则血气壅滞，故为烦躁，寝卧不得安宁。"指出凡是火邪扰动心神，心神不安，可致心烦失眠。

《素问玄机原病式•火类》说："躁动烦热，扰乱而不宁，火之体也。热甚于外，则肢体躁烦；热甚于内，则神志躁动。"指出心火内扰心神，神志不宁，可致躁动不安。

《诸病源候论•心病诸候》说："心与小肠合为表里，俱象于火，而火为阳气也。心为诸脏主，故正经不受邪，若为邪所伤而痛即死，若支别络脉为风邪所乘而痛，则经久成疹。其痛悬急懊者，是

邪迫于阳气，不得宣畅，壅瘀生热，故心如悬而急，烦懊痛也。"指
出心火扰动，心中悬急，可致心烦懊憹。

《血证论•脏腑病机论》说："火扰其血，则懊憹，神不清明则虚
烦不眠，动悸惊惕。"心主血脉，火扰其血，则是扰动心神，心神不
安，因而引起心烦懊憹，失眠惊悸等症。

《诸病源候论•心病候》说："心气盛，为神有余，…喜笑不休，
是心气之实也。"气有余便是火，心气盛则是心火亢盛，扰乱心神，
精神错乱，故引起喜笑不休。

《济生方•心小肠虚实论》说："及其实也，实则生热，热则心神
烦乱，面赤身热，…喜笑恐悸，其脉洪实，是实热之候也。"指出热
扰心神，可致心烦不宁，甚者可致精神错乱，喜笑不休。

《笔花医镜•心部》说："心之热，火迫之也，为烦躁，为不得
卧，为癫狂，为谵语。"指出实热扰神，心阳亢逆，而致神志错乱，
可引发各种精神狂越的病机。

7.1.2 Heat Falling into the Pericardium

After a person has contracted external warm heat disease evils, evil heat
can become exuberant. It may pass from the defense aspect to the qì aspect and then enter deeply into the construction and blood. Alternatively,
when warm evils are contracted in the upper body, they may first invade
the lungs and then pass abnormally to the pericardium. Both situations
are involved in the pathomechanisms of heat blocking the pericardium.

When heat enters the construction and blood and falls internally to
the pericardium, the pericardium catches the evil instead of the heart.
This results in intense heat in the interior, producing scorching heat and
blazing fire. Heat stimulates hyperactivity of heart yáng and the heat may
block the orifices of the heart. When the spirit light is driven by fire, the
heart spirit is harassed. This often manifests as a high fever with vexation
and agitation, unquiet sleep, or somnolence, possibly to the point of abnormalities of the spirit-mind.

Mild cases of heat falling into the pericardium result in clouded spirit
and delirious speech. Severe cases are marked by clouding and fretting with
an inability to speak, forward-staring eyes, and manic derangement. This
occurs because yáng heat is blocked internally and exuberant heat congests
the blood. The obstruction of qì and blood causes yáng qì to fail to move
outward to the network vessels of the tongue and the four limbs. This can
result in sluggishness of the tongue and reversal in the limbs. It should be
treated by clearing the heart and cooling construction while diffusing the
block and opening the orifices. For a formula, use Construction-Clearing

Decoction (*qīng yíng tāng*) in combination with Peaceful Palace Bovine Bezoar Pill (*ān gōng niú huáng wán*). These formulas are both from the *Wēn Bìng Tiáo Biàn* ("Systematized Identification of Warm Diseases").

Construction-Clearing Decoction (清营汤 *qīng yíng tāng*)
xī jiǎo (犀角 Rhinocerotis Cornu, rhinoceros horn)
lián qiào xīn (连翘心 Forsythiae Semen, forsythia seed)
zhú yè xīn (竹叶心 Lophatheri Folium Immaturum, tender lophatherum leaf)
lián zǐ xīn (莲子心 Nelumbinis Plumula, lotus plumule)
xuán shēn (玄参 Scrophulariae Radix, scrophularia)
mài dōng (麦冬 Ophiopogonis Radix, ophiopogon)

Peaceful Palace Bovine Bezoar Pill (安宫牛黄丸 *ān gōng niú huáng wán*)
niú huáng (牛黄 Bovis Calculus, bovine bezoar)
xī jiǎo (犀角 Rhinocerotis Cornu, rhinoceros horn)
yù jīn (郁金 Curcumae Radix, curcuma)
zhū shā (朱砂 Cinnabaris, cinnabar)
huáng lián (黄连 Coptidis Rhizoma, coptis)
huáng qín (黄芩 Scutellariae Radix, scutellaria)
zhī zǐ (栀子 Gardeniae Fructus, gardenia)
xióng huáng (雄黄 Realgar, realgar)
zhēn zhū (珍珠 Margarita, pearl)
shè xiāng (麝香 Moschus, musk)
bīng piàn (冰片 Borneolum, borneol)

热陷心包

外感温热病邪，邪热亢盛，由卫及气，深入营血；或温邪上受，首先犯肺，逆传心包，均可导致热闭心包的病机。热入营血，内陷心包，心包代心受邪，里热炽盛，热灼火燔，心阳为热激亢，心窍为热所闭，神明为火所逼，而致心神扰乱。常见高热烦躁，夜卧不安，嗜睡，进而引起神志异常。轻者神昏谵语，严重时昏愦不语，直视狂乱。同时因阳热内闭，热盛血壅，气血受阻，阳气不能运达舌络、四肢，可引起舌謇、肢厥。治宜清心凉营，宣闭开窍。方用《温病条辨》清宫汤（犀角尖、连翘心、竹叶心、莲子心、玄参心、麦冬）送服《温病条辨》安宫牛黄丸（牛黄、犀角、郁金、朱砂、黄连、黄芩、栀子、雄黄、珍珠、麝香、冰片）。

Literature Review of Heat Falling into the Pericardium

📖 *Wēn Rè Jīng Wěi* ("Warp and Weft of Warm Heat"), "Chapter by Yè Xiāng-Yán on Externally Contracted Warm Heat"

"If a disorder remains unresolved, it tends to gradually enter the construction. When the construction aspect contracts heat, the blood is robbed and the heart spirit becomes disquiet. This condition worsens at night and causes sleeplessness."

This quotation points out that warm heat evil qì normally invades the defense and qì aspects first, only afterwards entering the construction aspect. Since construction is linked to the heart, the normal passage of heat evil is to enter the pericardium.

📖 *Wēn Rè Jīng Wěi* ("Warp and Weft of Warm Heat"), "Chapter by Yè Xiāng-Yán on Externally Contracted Warm Heat"

"When warm evil is contracted in the upper body, it first invades the lungs before passing abnormally to the pericardium."

This quotation points out that warm heat evil qì can fall internally from the construction and qì aspects to pass abnormally to the pericardium.

📖 *Wēn Rè Jīng Wěi* ("Warp and Weft of Warm Heat"), "Chapter by Chén Píng-Bó on Externally Contracted Warm Heat"

"In cases of wind warmth patterns, the symptoms of heat effusion, thirst, oppression, and vexation, as well as clouding loss of consciousness, an inability to speak as if in a condition of deathlike reversal, and a rapid pulse are signs of internally brewing heat evils penetrating into the pericardium."

Another quotation:

"Extreme exuberance of heat evils fanning with the ministerial fire of the triple burner easily penetrates into the pericardium, driving the spirit light and blocking the network vessels. This will result in stupor and inability to speak with a corpse-like appearance."

These quotations both point out that evil heat that invades the pericardium and harasses the heart spirit can lead to clouding and fretting of the essence-spirit.

文献评述

《温热经纬•叶香岩外感温热篇》说："若病仍不解，是渐欲入营也，营分受热，则血液受劫，心神不安，夜甚无寐。"指出温热邪气一般是先侵犯卫分、气分，然后再入营分，营属心，热邪顺传可入心包。

《温热经纬•叶香岩外感温热篇》说："温邪上受，首先犯肺，逆传心包。"指出温热邪气也可以由卫气分内陷，逆传心包。

《温热经纬•陈平伯外感温热篇》说："风温证，热渴闷烦，昏愦不知人，不语如尸厥，脉数者，此热邪内蕴，走窜心包。"又说："热邪极盛，与三焦相火相煽，最易内窜心包，逼迫神明，闭塞络脉，以致昏迷不语，其状如尸。"均指出邪热侵犯心包，扰乱心神，可致精神昏愦。

7.1.3 Heat Entering the Heart Construction

When warm heat evil qì in the qì aspect enters deeper into the construction aspect, vigorous heat evil damages the construction yīn, concurrently damaging the yīn liquids. At the onset of night, defense yáng enters the interior from the exterior of the body and yáng qì enters yīn. On the one hand, this assists and extends evil heat; on the other hand, it exacerbates the damage to the yīn humor and the outward floating of yáng qì. Both of these factors increase the severity of nighttime heat effusion. Generalized heat effusion that worsens at night is typical of heat-type presentations.

During the qì aspect stage, vigorous heat damages the fluids, causing great thirst. After heat enters the heart construction, heat evil steams and soars into the blood and fluids, bearing upwards into the mouth. At this time, the patient will experience only slight thirst or no thirst at all. When heat evil enters deeply into the construction aspect and ascends to harass the heart, it disquiets the heart spirit and causes heart vexation, agitation, and insomnia.

When the condition is severe, evil heat will gradually spread to the heart spirit. This causes intermittent derangement of the heart spirit, which manifests as delirious speech and manic agitation. If heat evil scorches the sinew membranes of the liver channel, there is hypertonicity and tension. This results in upward staring eyes, rigidity of the neck, convulsions of the extremities, and arched-back rigidity. It should be treated by clearing construction and outthrusting heat while opening the orifices and extinguishing wind. For a formula, use Scourge-Clearing Toxin-Vanquishing Beverage (*qīng wēn bài dú yǐn*) from the *Yì Zhěn Yī Dé* ("A View of Epidemics Characterized by Papules"), with the addition of Peaceful Palace Bovine Bezoar Pill (*ān gōng niú huáng wán*) from the *Wēn Bìng Tiáo Biàn* ("Systematized Identification of Warm Diseases") (found in section 7.1.2) or Purple Snow Elixir (*zǐ xuě dān*) from the *Wēn Bìng Tiáo Biàn* ("Systematized Identification of Warm Diseases").

Scourge-Clearing Toxin-Vanquishing Beverage
(清瘟败毒饮 *qīng wēn bài dú yǐn*)

huáng lián (黄连 Coptidis Rhizoma, coptis)

huáng qín (黄芩 Scutellariae Radix, scutellaria)

zhī zǐ (栀子 Gardeniae Fructus, gardenia)

xī jiǎo (犀角 Rhinocerotis Cornu, rhinoceros horn)

shēng dì huáng (生地黄 Rehmanniae Radix Exsiccata seu Recens, dried/fresh rehmannia)

mǔ dān pí (牡丹皮 Moutan Cortex, moutan)

chì sháo (赤芍 Paeoniae Radix Rubra, red peony)

shí gāo (石膏 Gypsum Fibrosum, gypsum)

zhī mǔ (知母 Anemarrhenae Rhizoma, anemarrhena)

xuán shēn (玄参 Scrophulariae Radix, scrophularia)

dàn zhú yè (淡竹叶 Lophatheri Herba, lophatherum)

lián qiào (连翘 Forsythiae Fructus, forsythia)

jié gěng (桔梗 Platycodonis Radix, platycodon)

gān cǎo (甘草 Glycyrrhizae Radix, licorice)

Plus:

Peaceful Palace Bovine Bezoar Pill (安宫牛黄丸 *ān gōng niú huáng wán*)

Or:

Purple Snow Elixir (紫雪丹 *zǐ xuě dān*)

líng yáng jiǎo (羚羊角 Saigae Tataricae Cornu, antelope horn)

shí gāo (石膏 Gypsum Fibrosum, gypsum)

hán shuǐ shí (寒水石 Gypsum seu Calcitum, glauberite)

cí shí (磁石 Magnetitum, loadstone)

huá shí (滑石 Talcum, talcum)

"Heat entering the heart construction" refers to warm heat evil qì entering deeply into the construction aspect, where it scorches construction yīn. This pathomechanism manifests as the initial robbing of true yīn; the emphasis lies in the fact that construction yīn has been damaged. Since construction qì flows into the heart, damage to construction yīn spreads to harass and stir the heart spirit, resulting in heart vexation and insomnia. In cases where evil heat gradually ascends to intermittently harass the heart spirit, the symptoms of a clouded spirit and delirious speech also occur intermittently.

"Heat falling into the pericardium" refers to the direct invasion of the pericardium by warm heat evil qì. The key point of this pathomechanism is that after entering deeply into the heart, the evil contracted by the heart is taken on by the pericardium. Thus, the heart spirit is clouded, blocked, and distressed, leading to constant spirit clouding and delirious raving. In severe cases, when the movement of the blood becomes obstructed and the network vessels of the tongue and limbs are deprived of nourishment, it will result in sluggishness of the tongue and limb reversal.

Thus, there are definite differences between heat entering the heart construction and heat falling into the pericardium, both in terms of the sequence of disease locations, as well as in the severity of the pathological conditions.

热入心营

温热邪气由气分深入营分，壮热之邪伤及营阴，阴津同时受到损伤，到了夜晚，卫阳由表入里，阳气入阴，一方面助长邪热，另一方面更加重阴液的损伤，阳气外浮，均会使夜晚发热加重，引起身热夜重的典型热型。气分阶段，壮热伤津，口已大渴，热入心营后，热邪蒸腾血中津液，上承于口，此时表现为口不甚渴，或竟不渴。热邪深入营分而上扰于心，心神不安，而心烦躁扰，不能安睡；严重时，邪热渐接波及心神，阵阵引起心神错乱，则时而谵语狂躁。热邪灼伤肝经筋膜，筋膜挛急，则为两目上视，颈项强直，手足抽搐，角弓反张。治宜清营透热，开窍熄风。方用《疫疹一得》清温败毒饮（黄连、黄芩、栀子、犀角、生地、牡丹皮、赤芍、生石膏、知母、玄参、竹叶、连翘、桔梗、甘草）加《温病条辨》安宫牛黄丸或《温病条辨》紫雪丹（羚羊角、石膏、寒水石、磁石、滑石）。

热入心营是温热邪气深入营分，灼伤营阴，真阴初劫所表现的病机，重点在于营阴受损。由于营气通于心，当营阴受损时，波及并扰动心神，故而引起心烦不寐；邪热渐接上扰心神，时而干扰，故神昏谵语也是时而发生。热陷心包是温热邪气直接侵犯心包，病机重点已深入于心，心包代心受邪，心神为之蒙闭、逼迫，故而不断引起神昏谵妄，甚至血行受阻，舌络肢体失养，导致舌謇肢厥。因此热入心营与热陷心包在病位层次和病情轻重上均有一定差异。

Literature Review of Heat Entering the Heart Construction

📖 *Shāng Hán Zhǐ Zhǎng* ("A Guidebook on Cold Damage"), "Pathoconditions of Cold Damage"

"With regard to the construction aspect of the hand lesser yīn channel, if inhaled warm evils move from the defense to the construction, the patient's tongue will first be white and then turn crimson. Alternatively, if evils enter the construction aspect directly, the tongue will be crimson red or red with a slightly white center; this is accompanied by symptoms of nighttime vexation and insomnia, as well as torpid spirit and delirious speech."

This quotation explains that when heat evils enter construction and affect the heart, there may be heart vexation and insomnia, clouded spirit, and delirious speech.

📖 *Wēn Bìng Tiáo Biàn* ("Systematized Identification of Warm Diseases"), "Chapter on the Upper Burner"

"Summerheat-warmth in the hand reverting yīn channel will manifest as generalized heat effusion without an aversion to cold, an unclear spirit, and intermittent delirious speech."

This quotation points out that when summerheat-heat invades construction blood, it chaotically drives the heart spirit, resulting in spirit clouding and delirious speech.

📖 *Wēn Bìng Tiáo Biàn* ("Systematized Identification of Warm Diseases"), "Chapter on the Upper Burner"

"In greater yīn warm diseases, the inch pulse is large, the tongue is crimson and dry, and the patient should suffer from thirst. If there is no thirst, this means that the heat is located in the construction aspect; Construction-Clearing Decoction (*qīng yíng tāng*) without coptis governs. Thirst is a fundamental sign of warm disease. In the present case, the absence of thirst can mislead people in spite of the fact that the symptoms of a crimson and dry tongue and a large inch pulse are associated with warm disease. The absence of thirst results because evil heat entering the construction aspect steams and soars up, causing construction qì to ascend"

This quotation explains that if heat evil enters the construction aspect, it steams and soars, causing construction yīn to ascend. This pathomechanism does not produce great thirst.

文献评述

《伤寒指掌•伤寒类症》："手少阴营分，温邪吸入，由卫及营者，其舌先白后绛也。或竟入营分，则舌必绛赤，或红中兼微白，夜烦不寐，神呆谵语。"说明热邪入营，波及于心，可致心烦不寐，神昏谵语。

《温病条辨•上焦篇》说："手厥阴暑温，身热不恶寒，清神不了了，时时谵语。"指出暑热侵入营血，逼乱心神，可致神昏谵语。

《温病条辨•上焦篇》说："太阴温病，寸脉大，舌绛而干，法当渴，今反不渴者，热在营中也，清营汤去黄连主之。渴乃温之本病，今乃不渴，滋人疑惑，而舌绛且干，寸脉大，的系温病。盖邪热入营蒸腾，营气上升，故不渴。"充分说明热邪入营，蒸腾营阴上升，可致口不甚渴的病机。

<table>
<tr><td colspan="1" align="center">Summary of Evil Heat Harassing the Spirit</td></tr>
</table>

1. Heart Fire Harassing the Spirit
   Mild patterns: Heart palpitations, heart vexation, heat and oppression in the chest, anguish, tossing and turning, insomnia and profuse dreaming
   Severe patterns: Agitation, vexation, derangement, clouded spirit and delirious speech, incessant laughing.
2. Heat Falling into the Pericardium
   High fever, vexation and agitation, unquiet sleep, somnolence, clouded spirit and delirious speech, clouding and fretting with an inability to speak, forward-staring eyes and manic derangement, a sluggish tongue, and limb reversal
3. Heat Entering the Heart Construction
   Generalized heat effusion that worsens at night, absence of severe thirst or no thirst at all, heart vexation and agitation, unquiet sleep; at times possibly delirious speech and manic agitation, staring upward of the eyes, rigidity of the neck, convulsions of the extremities, and arched-back rigidity

---

邪热扰神

心火扰神
　　轻证 —— 心悸心烦，胸中热闷，懊憹颠倒，失眠多梦。
　　重证 —— 躁动烦乱，神昏谵语，喜笑不休。
热陷心包
　　高热烦躁，夜卧不安，嗜睡。神昏谵语，昏愦不语，直视狂乱。舌謇、肢厥。
热入心营
　　身热夜甚，口不甚渴，或竟不渴。心烦躁扰，夜卧不安，时或谵语狂躁。两目上视，颈项强直，手足抽搐，角弓反张。

7.2 Phlegm Fire Harassing the Heart

Several situations can result in the mutual binding of phlegm and fire. Damage by the seven affects causes qì depression and the formation of phlegm; depressed phlegm may transform into fire. Alternatively, excess among the five minds can cause fire formation, and fire or heat can scorch the fluids and condense the humors into phlegm. In the case of externally contracted heat disorders, exuberant heat scorches the fluids and condenses them into phlegm.

When there is internal exuberance of phlegm and fire, they contend with and strike at each other. In the *Zhèng Zhì Huì Bǔ* ("A Supplement to Patterns and Treatment"), "Phlegm Patterns," it states, "Phlegm, encountering fire, boils and soars up; fire, encountering phlegm, fans intensely." This forms a pathomechanism of phlegm and fire binding together. Phlegm easily causes clouding while fire easily causes distress. When phlegm clouds the orifices of the heart, the spirit becomes ungoverned, resulting in clouding and fretting. When fire drives the spirit light, there is derangement and frenetic movement of the essence-spirit.

At times of mild harassment from phlegm and fire, the heart is harassed and unquiet, which frequently manifests in such symptoms as heart vexation, insomnia, and profuse dreaming. In the daytime, there may be cumbersome fatigue with a desire to sleep but an inability to fall asleep. Night brings an increase in mental activity without the slightest sign of drowsiness; this is a sign of stirring and floating of the heart spirit. Suitable treatment involves clearing heat and eliminating phlegm while draining fire and quieting the spirit. For a formula, choose a modified version of Coptis Gallbladder-Warming Decoction (*huáng lián wēn dǎn tāng*) from the *Liù Yīn Tiáo Biàn* ("Identification According to the Six Causes").

Coptis Gallbladder-Warming Decoction (黄连温胆汤 *huáng lián wēn dǎn tāng*)
huáng lián (黄连 Coptidis Rhizoma, coptis)
bàn xià (半夏 Pinelliae Rhizoma, pinellia)
fú líng (茯苓 Poria, poria)
chén pí (陈皮 Citri Reticulatae Pericarpium, tangerine peel)
zhǐ qiào (*ké*) (枳壳 Aurantii Fructus, bitter orange)
zhú rú (竹茹 Bumbusae Caulis in Taenia, bamboo shavings)
gān cǎo (甘草 Glycyrrhizae Radix, licorice)
shēng jiāng (生姜 Zingiberis Rhizoma Recens, fresh ginger)

When phlegm fire is rampant, the heart spirit is harassed and the spirit light becomes clouded and deranged, resulting in the following symptoms: manic agitation, frenetic stirring, mania with sudden loss of consciousness, disordered speech, abnormal laughing and crying, cursing, yelling, and hitting people and smashing objects regardless of who is present. Suitable treatment involves flushing phlegm and downbearing fire while opening the orifices and quieting the spirit. For a formula, choose

Chlorite/Mica Phlegm-Rolling Pill (*méng shí gǔn tán wán*) from the *Dān Xī Xīn Fǎ Fù Yú* ("A Supplement to Dān-Xī's Heart-Approach"), in combination with Two Matured Ingredients Decoction (*èr chén tāng*) from the *Tài Píng Huì Mín Hé Jì Jú Fāng* ("Tài-Píng Imperial Grace Pharmacy Formulas"), with the addition of coptis, bile arisaema, and aquilaria.

Chlorite/Mica Phlegm-Rolling Pill (礞石滚痰丸 *méng shí gǔn tán wán*)
méng shí (礞石 Chloriti seu Micae Lapis, chlorite/mica)
huáng qín (黄芩 Scutellariae Radix, scutellaria)
dà huáng (大黄 Rhei Radix et Rhizoma, rhubarb)
chén xiāng (沉香 Aquilariae Lignum Resinatum, aquilaria)

Two Matured Ingredients Decoction (二陈汤 *èr chén tāng*)
bàn xià (半夏 Pinelliae Rhizoma, pinellia)
jú hóng (橘红 Citri Reticulatae Pericarpium Rubrum, red tangerine peel)
fú líng (茯苓 Poria, poria)
zhì gān cǎo (炙甘草 Glycyrrhizae Radix cum Liquido Fricta, mix-fried licorice)
shēng jiāng (生姜 Zingiberis Rhizoma Recens, fresh ginger)
wū méi (乌梅 Mume Fructus, mume)
Plus:
huáng lián (黄连 Coptidis Rhizoma, coptis)
dǎn xīng (胆星 Arisaema cum Bile, bile arisaema)
chén xiāng (沉香 Aquilariae Lignum Resinatum, aquilaria)

痰火扰心

七情所伤，气郁生痰，痰郁化火；或五志化火，火热灼津，炼液为痰；或外感热病，热盛灼津，炼液为痰，均能引起痰火互结为患。痰火内盛，互相搏击，"痰得火而沸腾，火得痰而煽炽"（《证治汇补•痰证》），形成痰火交结的病机。痰易蒙蔽，火易逼迫，痰蒙心窍，神无所主而昏愦；火逼神明，精神错乱而妄动。痰火轻扰之时，心被扰而不宁，多见心烦不安、失眠多梦，白天困倦思眠，但不能入睡，夜间精神倍增，无丝毫睡意等心神浮动之象。治宜清热除痰，泻火安神。方选《六因条辨》黄连温胆汤（黄连、半夏、茯苓、陈皮、枳壳、竹茹、甘草、生姜）加减；痰火鸱张时，扰乱心神，神明昏乱，则为狂躁妄动、狂暴无知、语言杂乱、哭笑无常、骂詈叫号、打人毁物、不避亲疏等症。治宜涤痰降火，开窍安神。方选《丹溪心法附余》礞石滚痰丸（青礞石、黄芩、大黄、沉香）合《太平惠民和剂局方》二陈汤（半夏、橘红、茯苓、炙甘草、生姜、乌梅）加黄连、胆星、沉香。

Literature Review of Phlegm Fire Harassing the Heart

📖 *Jīng Yuè Quán Shū* ("Jǐng-Yuè's Complete Compendium"), "Schema of Miscellaneous Patterns," Section on "Withdrawal, Mania, and Feeble-mindedness"

"All manic disorders are predominantly caused by fire. This may result from making of strategies causing loss of mind or from thought and preoccupation causing depression and binding. There is bending without stretching and anger that is not vented, resulting in counterflow of liver and gallbladder qì. This is the combined evil of wood and fire, which is precisely the condition of Eastern Repletion Pattern. When the heart is overwhelmed by evil, the spirit and ethereal soul will fail to keep their composure."

This quotation points out that phlegm generated by qì depression may transform into fire and harass the heart spirit, leading to manic derangement.

📖 *Zhèng Zhì Huì Bǔ* ("A Supplement to Patterns and Treatment"), "Withdrawal and Mania"

"Mania is caused by phlegm fire adhering solidly to the heart and chest. It is an extreme yáng evil that may suddenly cause furious mania, as if possessed by spirits."

Again it states:

"Withdrawal is caused by heart fire. Heat amassment in the heart channel emerges irregularly; at times there may be vexation and agitation, a sensation of hot qì in the nose and eyes, and an inability to act freely. This condition is classified as heart wind and recurs after brief moments of stability. The formula Heart-Clearing Decoction (*qīng xīn tāng*) is appropriate, with the addition of acorus and possibly scutellaria, coptis, trichosanthes root, root poria, ophiopogon, salvia, polygala, and bovine bezoar."

From this quotation, it is clear that fire and phlegm are the primary etiological factors that cause harassment of the heart spirit. Fire often invades the heart spirit on its own; it may be identified in the qì aspect or in the construction, in both mild disorders as well as serious disorders. Fire can easily combine with phlegm to cloud and harass the heart spirit. The binding of phlegm and fire is difficult to resolve.

文献评述

《景岳全书·杂证谟·癫狂痴呆》说："凡狂病多因于火，此或以谋为失志，或以思虑郁结，屈无所伸，怒无所泄，以致肝胆气逆，木火合邪，是诚东方实证也，此其邪乘于心，则为神魂不守。"指出气郁生痰化火，扰乱心神，可致狂乱。

《证治汇补•癫狂》说："狂由痰火胶固心胸，阳邪充极，故猖狂刚暴，若有神灵所附。"又说："癫因心火：有心经蓄热，发作不常，或时烦躁，鼻眼觉有热气，不能自由，有类心风，稍定复作，宜<u>清心汤</u>，加菖蒲，或芩、连、花粉、茯神、麦冬、丹参、远志、牛黄之类。"由此可见，火、痰是引起心神受扰的主要因素。火常单独侵犯心神，有在气、在营，病轻、病重之辨，更易与痰相合，蒙蔽扰乱心神，胶结难解。

Summary of Phlegm Fire Harassing the Heart

1. Mild Harassment by Phlegm Fire
   Heart vexation, insomnia, profuse dreaming, cumbersome fatigue and a desire to sleep during the day with increased mental activity at night
2. Rampant Phlegm Fire
   Manic agitation, frenetic stirring, sudden mania, loss of consciousness, disordered speech, cursing, yelling, and hitting people and smashing objects regardless of who is present

痰火扰心
痰火轻扰 —— 心烦不安、失眠多梦，白天困倦思眠，夜间精神倍增。
痰火鸱张 —— 狂躁妄动、狂暴无知、语言杂乱、骂詈叫号、打人毁物、不避亲疏。

7.3　Heat Hurrying the Blood in the Vessels

The heart governs the blood vessels and heart yáng has the function of propelling the movement of blood. When the yáng qì of the heart is regulated and harmonized, the movement of blood is calm and leisurely, harmonious and moderate. If the heart is invaded by warm heat evil qì or if the yáng qì of the heart tends towards exuberance, fire and heat will be engendered internally. This affects the blood and manifests as thin flow in the vessels. The pathomechanisms involved here are frenetic movement of blood and heat putrefying the blood.

热迫血脉

心主血脉，心阳有推动血行之用。心的阳气调和，则血液运行从容和缓。若受温热邪气侵犯，或心的阳气偏盛，火热内生，作用于血，则易表现为脉流薄疾，迫血妄行和热腐血败等病机。

7.3.1   Thin Flow in the Vessels

In externally contracted heat disorders, heat enters the construction-blood. Consumption of excessive amounts of acrid, spicy, and stimulating foods causes heat evil to attack the heart. Alternatively, diseases of miscellaneous internal damage can cause hyperactivity of heart yáng. All these factors can lead to exuberant heat in the blood. Powerful heat shakes and arouses the heart viscus, forcing the heartbeat to accelerate. This can result in heart palpitations and a racing heartbeat. The distressed movement of blood, the accelerated pulse rate, and the pounding in the vessels can result in a pulse that is surging, replete, slippery, or rapid. It should be treated by clearing the heart and draining fire. For a formula, use Heart-Draining Decoction (*xiè xīn tāng*) from the *Jīn Guì Yào Lüè* ("Essential Prescriptions of the Golden Coffer").

Heart-Draining Decoction (泻心汤 *xiè xīn tāng*)

dà huáng (大黄 Rhei Radix et Rhizoma, rhubarb)
huáng lián (黄连 Coptidis Rhizoma, coptis)
huáng qín (黄芩 Scutellariae Radix, scutellaria)

脉流薄疾

外感热病，热入营血；过服辛辣刺激食物，热邪攻心；或内伤杂病，心阳偏亢，均会引起血热过盛。热势汹涌，振荡心脏，逼迫心跳加速，可致心悸悸动不宁；逼迫血行，加速脉率，冲击脉管，可致脉搏洪实滑数。治宜清心泻火，方用《金匮要略》泻心汤。

Literature Review of Thin Flow in the Vessels

📖 *Mài Jīng* ("The Pulse Canon"), "Disease Patterns of the Hand Lesser Yīn Channel"

"In heart disease…the face is red and the body is hot; the pulse is replete, large, and rapid."

This quotation points out that heart fire that distresses the blood and accelerates its movement can result in a pulse that is rapid.

📖 *Bǐ Huā Yī Jìng* ("*Bǐ Huā* Medical Mirror"), "Section on the Heart"

"Heat in the heart refers to distress from fire. The pulse will invariably be rapid in the left inch position."

The left inch position is ascribed to the heart. Heart fire forces the blood to flow more quickly. Therefore, one will observe a rapid pulse.

文献评述

《脉经•手少阴经病证》说："心病，…面赤身热，其脉实大而数。"指出心火逼迫，加快血行，可致脉数。

《笔花医镜•心部》说："心之热，火迫之也，脉左寸必数。"左寸属心，心火逼迫，血流增快，故见数脉。

7.3.2 Frenetic Movement of Blood

Exuberant heat in the blood may be caused by heat evils entering the blood. In addition to accelerating the blood flow, steaming and soaring heat in the blood can force the blood to move frenetically, causing it to surge and break the blood network vessels. This causes the blood to spill out of the vessels, resulting in a variety of acute bleeding patterns, such as blood ejection and spontaneous external bleeding.

Frenetic movement of blood manifests as bleeding with a fierce, turbulent onset, and is characterized by large amounts of blood loss; the blood has a fresh red color and the bleeding is difficult to stanch. It should be treated by clearing the heart and draining fire while cooling the blood and stanching bleeding. For a formula, use Red-Abducting Powder (*dǎo chì sǎn*) from the *Xiǎo Ér Yào Zhèng Zhí Jué* ("Key to Diagnosis and Treatment of Children's Diseases"), with the addition of imperata root, lotus root node, water buffalo horn, and agrimony.

Red-Abducting Powder (导赤散 *dǎo chì sǎn*)

shēng dì huáng (生地黄 Rehmanniae Radix Exsiccata seu Recens, dried/fresh rehmannia)

mù tōng (木通 Akebiae Trifoliatae Caulis, trifoliate akebia)

dàn zhú yè (淡竹叶 Lophatheri Herba, lophatherum)

gān cǎo (甘草 Glycyrrhizae Radix, licorice)

Plus:

bái máo gēn (白茅根 Imperatae Rhizoma, imperata)

ǒu jié (藕节 Nelumbinis Rhizomatis Nodus, lotus root node)

shuǐ niú jiǎo (水牛角 Bubali Cornu, water buffalo horn)

xiān hè cǎo (仙鹤草 Agrimoniae Herba, agrimony)

迫血妄行

邪热入血，血热亢盛，除加速血流外，还可因血热蒸腾，迫血妄行，冲破血络，溢出脉外，引起吐血、衄血等多种急性出血证。表现为来势汹猛，出血量多，血色鲜红，不易休止。治宜清心泻火，凉血止血。方用《小儿药证直诀》<u>导赤散</u>（生地、木通、竹叶、甘草）加白茅根、藕节、水牛角、仙鹤草。

Literature Review of Frenetic Movement of Blood

📖 *Zhū Bìng Yuán Hòu Lùn* ("The Origin and Indicators of Disease"), "Symptoms of Cold Damage with Spontaneous External Bleeding"

"The heart governs the blood and the liver stores the blood. When heat evil damages the heart or liver, it will cause spontaneous external bleeding."

This quotation points out that heat evil that damages the heart and forces the blood to move frenetically may result in spontaneous external bleeding.

📖 *Tài Píng Huì Mín Hé Jì Jú Fāng* ("Tài-Píng Imperial Grace Pharmacy Formulas"), "Various Formulas for Treating Incessant Blood Ejection"

"The condition of incessant blood ejection is caused by an accumulation of heat in the heart and lungs."

This quotation points out that when heat harasses the heart blood, exuberant heat will stir the blood and cause it to emerge in the upper body, possibly resulting in blood ejection. When it exits from the blood network vessels in the skin or muscles, it can cause macules or papules on the skin. From a clinical perspective, there are numerous factors that can cause bleeding; however, heart heat forcing the blood to move frenetically is one of the most important pathomechanisms.

文献评述

《诸病源候论•伤寒衄血候》说："心主于血，肝藏于血，热邪伤于心肝，故衄血也。"指出热邪伤心，迫血妄行，可致衄血。

《太平圣惠方•治吐血不止诸方》说："夫吐血不止者，由心肺积热。"指出热扰心血，热盛动血，从上而出，可致吐血；从皮肤血络或肌肉而出，致皮肤斑疹。临床上引起出血的原因很多，但心热迫血是最重要的病机之一。

7.3.3 Heat Putrefying the Blood

The *Sù Wèn* ("Plain Questions") text, in the "Great Treatise on the Essentials of Supreme Truth," states, "All painful and itching sores are ascribed to the heart." The heart governs the blood; if there is exuberant heart yáng and scorching from intense heart fire, the exuberant heat will wear on the blood and damage liquids. This reduces the fluids in the blood, causing the blood to become concentrated, thick, and sticky.

When the movement of blood gradually slows down and the blood becomes congested, the blood will collect, congeal, and bind; this results in swelling and distention. This condition leads to red painful swelling and the eruption of sores. The prolonged brewing of heat evil putrefies the flesh and vanquishes the blood, manifesting with swollen and suppurating welling-abscesses. It should be treated by draining fire and resolving toxins while dispersing swelling and expelling pus. For a formula, use Coptis Toxin-Resolving Decoction (*huáng lián jiě dú tāng*) from the *Wài Tái Mì Yào* ("Essential Secrets from Outside the Metropolis"), in combination with Immortal Formula Life-Giving Beverage (*xiān fāng huó mìng yǐn*) from the *Fù Rén Liáng Fāng* ("Good Remedies for Women").

Coptis Toxin-Resolving Decoction (黄连解毒汤 *huáng lián jiě dú tāng*)

huáng lián (黄连 Coptidis Rhizoma, coptis)
huáng qín (黄芩 Scutellariae Radix, scutellaria)
huáng bǎi (黄柏 Phellodendri Cortex, phellodendron)
zhī zǐ (栀子 Gardeniae Fructus, gardenia)

Immortal Formula Life-Giving Beverage
(仙方活命饮 *xiān fāng huó mìng yǐn*)

chuān shān jiǎ (穿山甲 Manis Squama, pangolin scales)
zào jiǎo cì (皂角刺 Gleditsiae Spina, gleditsia thorn)
tiān huā fěn (天花粉 Trichosanthis Radix, trichosanthes root)
jīn yín huā (金银花 Lonicerae Flos, lonicera)
dāng guī (当归 Angelicae Sinensis Radix, Chinese angelica)
chì sháo (赤芍 Paeoniae Radix Rubra, red peony)
rǔ xiāng (乳香 Olibanum, frankincense)
mò yào (没药 Myrrha, myrrh)
bái zhǐ (白芷 Angelicae Dahuricae Radix, Dahurian angelica)
fáng fēng (防风 Saposhnikoviae Radix, saposhnikovia)
bèi mǔ (贝母 Fritillariae Bulbus, fritillaria)
chén pí (陈皮 Citri Reticulatae Pericarpium, tangerine peel)
gān cǎo (甘草 Glycyrrhizae Radix, licorice)

热腐血败

《素问•至真要大论》说：“诸痛痒疮，皆属于心。”心主血，心阳亢盛，心火灼炽，热盛可耗血伤津，血中津液减少，血液浓缩粘稠，运行逐渐迟慢，血液壅阻、停滞、凝结、肿胀，引起红肿疼痛，则发为疮疡。热邪煎熬日久，肉腐血败，则会出现痛肿化脓。治宜泻火解毒，消肿排脓。方用《外台秘要》黄连解毒汤（黄连、黄芩、黄柏、栀子）合《妇人良方》仙方活命饮（穿山甲、皂角刺、天花粉、金银花、当归、赤芍、乳香、没药、白芷、防风、贝母、陈皮、甘草）。

Literature Review of Heat Putrefying the Blood

📖 *Lèi Jīng* ("The Classified Canon"), Scroll 13, commentary:

> "Severe heat results in painful sores; slight heat results in itchy sores. The heart is ascribed to fire and is involved in the formation of heat. Therefore, all sores are ascribed to the heart."

This quotation explains that exuberant heart fire is an important pathomechanism involved in the formation of swollen painful sores.

📖 *Líng Shū* ("The Magic Pivot"), "Chapter on Welling- and Flat-Abscesses"

> "Construction and defense flow continuously in the blood and vessels. … Exuberant heat putrefies the flesh and putrid flesh leads to pus."

This quotation sets forth the pathomechanisms involved in the generation of pus. Pus is formed from severe heat causing sores to become putrefied.

文献评述

《类经》十三卷注曰："热甚则疮痛，热微则疮痒，心属火，其化热，故疮疡皆属于心也。"说明心火亢盛，是形成疮疡肿痛的重要病机。

《灵枢·痈疽篇》说："夫血脉营卫，周流不休，……热盛则腐肉，肉腐则为脓。"阐述了热甚可使疮疡腐败，化生脓液的病机。

Summary of Heat Hurrying the Movement of Blood

1. Thin Flow in the Vessels
   Shaking the Heart: Heart palpitations
   Accelerated Movement of the Blood: A pulse that is surging, replete, slippery, and/or rapid
2. Frenetic Movement of the Blood
   Blood ejection or spontaneous external bleeding with a turbulent and fierce onset; the bleeding is in large quantities, the blood is fresh red in color, and the bleeding is difficult to stanch
3. Heat Putrefying the Blood
   Eruption of red swollen painful sores, possibly manifesting with welling-abscesses and pus

热迫血行
脉流薄疾 　　振荡心体 —— 心悸悸动。 　　加快血行 —— 脉搏洪实滑数。 迫血妄行 　　吐血、衄血，来势汹猛，出血量多，血色鲜红，不易休止。 热腐血败 　　红肿疼痛，发为疮疡，出现痈脓。

7.4　Heart Fire Flaming Upward and Spreading Downward

Repletion heat in the heart channel may refer to heat harassing the heart spirit, phlegm fire harassing the heart, or heat hurrying the blood in the vessels. In addition, when yáng heat is exuberant, intense internal heart fire may be conveyed upward or downward along the heart channel. This tends to manifest in two primary ways: upward flaming or downward spreading of heart fire.

上炎下移

心经实热，除热扰心神，痰火扰心，热迫血脉外，当阳热亢盛，心火内炽时，可沿心经经脉上下传变，出现上炎和下移两大趋势。

7.4.1　Upward Flaming of Heart Fire

The heart governs the blood and vessels and has its bloom in the face. Thus, changes in the color and sheen of the face are external indicators of the exuberance or debility of qì and blood. The heart is also involved with the tongue; it is said that the heart opens at the tongue and the tongue is the sprout of the heart. In addition, the divergent channel of the heart ascends to tie at the root of the tongue.

When heart yáng is hyperactive and heart fire is intensely exuberant, the fire may be fixed along the heart channel. If fire comes into contact with blood heat to flame and steam upwards, it may manifest in numerous types of repletion fire patterns affecting the head and face.

When heart fire ascends to harass the face, the blood vessels of the face will be full and blood heat will be exuberant, manifesting in patterns with red eyes, redness of the whole face, and sores on the face. Heart fire that ascends to harass the mouth and tongue will manifest with exuberant heat and congested blood. Heat that putrefies the blood will engender sores of the mouth and tongue, as well as erosion, swelling, and pain.

Additional patterns affecting the tongue may be observed, such as a red-tipped tongue, swelling of the tongue, spontaneous bleeding of the tongue, protrusion or worrying of the tongue, or a double tongue. It should be treated by clearing the heart and draining fire. For a formula, use Red-Abducting Powder (*dǎo chì sǎn*) from the text *Xiǎo Ér Yào Zhèng Zhí Jué* ("Key to Diagnosis and Treatment of Children's Diseases"), with the addition of coptis, scutellaria, and forsythia.

Red-Abducting Powder (导赤散 *dǎo chì sǎn*)

shēng dì huáng (生地黄 Rehmanniae Radix Exsiccata seu Recens, dried/fresh rehmannia)
mù tōng (木通 Akebiae Trifoliatae Caulis, trifoliate akebia)
dàn zhú yè (淡竹叶 Lophatheri Herba, lophatherum)
gān cǎo (甘草 Glycyrrhizae Radix, licorice)
Plus:
huáng lián (黄连 Coptidis Rhizoma, coptis)
huáng qín (黄芩 Scutellariae Radix, scutellaria)
lián qiào (连翘 Forsythiae Fructus, forsythia)

心火上炎

心主血脉，其华在面，面部色泽变化为气血盛衰的外部标志。心开窍于舌，舌乃心之苗。心经之别上系舌本，故当心阳偏亢，心火炽盛时，火势沿着心经经脉，或通过血热向上炎蒸，表现头面多种实火见症。心火上扰于面，面部血脉充盈，血热亢盛，则见目睛红赤、满面通红、面部疮疡等症。心火上扰口舌，热盛血壅，热腐血败，则为口舌生疮、糜烂肿痛，或见舌尖红赤、舌肿、舌衄、吐舌弄舌、重舌等症。治宜清心泻火。方用《小儿药证直诀》导赤散加黄连、黄芩、连翘。

Literature Review of Upward Flaming of Heart Fire

📖 *Sù Wèn* ("Plain Questions"), "On Wilting"

 "Heart heat manifests in a red complexion and spillage from the vessels."

This quotation points out that upward flaming of heart fire and ascendant counterflow of qì and blood cause the blood vessels of the face to become full, resulting in a red face and red eyes.

📖 *Sù Wèn* ("Plain Questions"), "Great Treatise on the Essentials of Supreme Truth"

 "Heat in the heart causes vexation and agitation...Fire qì arises internally and ascends to cause oral putrescence, retching counterflow, and blood spillage or blood discharge."

This quotation points out that heart qì attacking the upper body causes exuberant heat, blood congestion, and heat putrefying the blood. This results in ulceration and sores of the mouth and tongue.

📖 *Jì Shēng Fāng* ("Formulas for Saving Lives"), "On the Treatment of Heart and Small Intestine Vacuity and Repletion"

> "Repletion leads to the generation of heat. Heat leads to vexation and derangement of the heart spirit, a red face and generalized heat effusion, and the formation of mouth and tongue sores."

This quotation points out that heart fire harassing the upper body can result in signs such as a red face and eyes or mouth and tongue sores.

📖 *Zhū Bìng Yuán Hòu Lùn* ("The Origin and Indicators of Disease")

In "Symptoms of Bleeding from the Upper Surface of the Tongue," it states:

> "The heart governs the blood and vessels and manifests its symptoms in the tongue. If there is heat in the heart viscus, blood will emerge from the upper surface of the tongue like a gushing spring."

Another quote from the chapter, "Symptoms of Sores of the Mouth and Tongue" states:

> "The hand lesser yīn is the channel of the heart. The flow of heart qì reaches the tongue. … In cases with exuberant heat in the viscera and bowels, heat overwhelms the heart and spleen. This causes qì to surge into the mouth and tongue, leading to the formation of mouth and tongue sores."

In the chapter "Symptoms of a Double Tongue," it states:

> "When there is heat present in the heart or spleen, heat qì follows the vessels and surges into the root of the tongue. The blood vessels become distended and change to form a tongue-shaped form that is located below the root of the tongue. This is called a double tongue."

These quotes elaborate the different changes in the shape of the tongue that can result from either upward flaming of heart fire to the orifice of the tongue, hurried blood, binding of heat, or surging of heat.

📖 *Xuè Zhèng Lùn* ("Treatise on Blood Patterns"), "On the Pathomechanisms of the Bowels and Viscera"

> "The heart vessel ascends along the throat and nets the root of the tongue. Repletion fire congesting in the upper body results in throat impediment. Ascending vacuity fire causes stiffness of the tongue and an inability to speak."

Here Mr. Wáng points out that heart fire can lead to pathological changes in the throat, mouth, and tongue when it follows its channel to harass the upper body.

文献评述

《素问•痿论》说："心热者，色赤而脉络溢。"指出心火上炎，气血上逆，面部血脉充盈，可致面目红赤。

《素问•至真要大论》说："心热烦躁，……火气内发，上为口糜呕逆，血溢血泄。"指出心热上攻，热盛血壅，热腐血败，可致口舌溃烂生疮。

《济生方•心小肠虚实论治》：说"及其实也，实则生热，热则心神烦乱，面赤身热，口舌生疮。"指出心火上扰，可致面目红赤，口舌生疮等症。

《诸病源候论•舌上出血候》说："心主血脉，而候于舌，若心脏有热，则舌上出血如涌泉。"《口舌疮候》又说："手少阴，心之经也，心气通于舌。……脏腑热盛，热乘心脾，气冲于口与舌，故令口舌生疮也。"《重舌候》亦说："心脾有热，热气随脉冲于舌本，血脉胀起，变生如舌之状，在于舌本之下，谓之重舌。"均阐述了心火上炎舌窍，或迫血、或热结、或热冲可引起各种舌形改变。

《血证论•脏腑病机论》说："心之脉上挟咽喉，络于舌本，实火上壅为喉痹，虚火上升则舌强不能言。"

王氏也指出心火沿经脉上扰，可引起咽喉、口舌的病变。

7.4.2   Fire Spreading Downward to the Small Intestine

The heart and small intestine are linked in an interior-exterior relationship. The hand lesser yīn channel originates in the center of the heart and descends to net the small intestine. When heart yáng is exuberant and heart fire flames upward, it can also simultaneously follow its channel to spread downward to the small intestine. The decocting of heat evil causes the small intestine to be unable to separate the clear and turbid. Thus, fluids cannot be transported down to the bladder and there will be poor bladder qì transformation.

This condition manifests with red or yellow urine, hot or painful urination, or possibly stagnant, rough, inhibited urination. When heat damages the blood network vessels and forces blood to spill out, it can manifest as bloody urination. This condition should be treated by clearing the heart and draining fire while freeing the small intestine. For a formula, use Red-Abducting Powder (*dǎo chì sǎn*) from the *Xiǎo Ér Yào Zhèng Zhí Jué* ("Key to Diagnosis and Treatment of Children's Diseases"), with the addition of coptis, fried gardenia, moutan, field thistle, and knotgrass.

Red-Abducting Powder (导赤散 *dǎo chì sǎn*)

shēng dì huáng (生地黄 Rehmanniae Radix Exsiccata seu Recens, dried/fresh rehmannia)

mù tōng (木通 Akebiae Trifoliatae Caulis, trifoliate akebia)

dàn zhú yè (淡竹叶 Lophatheri Herba, lophatherum)

gān cǎo (甘草 Glycyrrhizae Radix, licorice)

Plus:

huáng lián (黄连 Coptidis Rhizoma, coptis)

zhī zǐ (栀子 Gardeniae Fructus, gardenia)

mǔ dān pí (牡丹皮 Moutan Cortex, moutan)

xiǎo jì (小蓟 Cirsii Herba, field thistle)

biǎn xù (萹蓄 Polygoni Avicularis Herba, knotgrass)

心与小肠互为表里，手少阴之脉，起于心中，下络小肠。当心阳亢盛，心火上炎之际，同时又可沿其经脉下移小肠。热邪煎熬，小肠不能泌别清浊，津液不能下输膀胱，膀胱气化不行，则见小便黄赤、尿热尿痛、滞涩不畅；热伤血络，迫血外溢，则为尿血。治宜清心泻火，通利小肠。方用《小儿药证直诀》导赤散加黄连、炒栀、丹皮、小蓟、萹蓄。

Literature Review of Fire Spreading Downward to the Small Intestine

📖 *Sù Wèn* ("Plain Questions"), "On Wilting"

"Excessive sorrow and grief causes the expiry of the pericardiac network. Expiry of the pericardiac network results in internal stirring of yáng qì and flooding below the heart, along with frequent bloody urination."

The pericardiac network constitutes the external defense of the heart. Yáng qì stirs internally because of exuberant heart fire, giving rise to urinary frequency and bloody urine. This is caused by the fact that the heart and small intestine are interconnected, which allows heart fire to spread downward to the small intestine.

📖 *Zhū Bìng Yuán Hòu Lùn* ("The Origin and Indicators of Disease"), "The Symptoms of Blood Disorders"

"The heart governs the blood and is connected to the small intestine. If heat is present in the abode of the heart, it will bind in the small intestine, causing bloody urine."

This clearly points out that heat in the heart channel can be transmitted down the channel to spread into the small intestine. This forces the blood to move frenetically and leads to bloody urination.

📖 *Jĭng Yuè Quán Shū* ("Jĭng-Yuè's Complete Compendium"), "Schema of Miscellaneous Patterns, Blood Patterns"

"Blood found in the urine hole [urinary meatus] originally comes from the small intestine. In this pattern, the urine hole does not hurt, but blood emerges following the urine, possibly with dull pain in the navel and abdomen or signs of heat in the bowels and viscera. The small intestine and the heart are linked in an exterior-interior relationship. This is the source of qì transformation in the third heavenly stem of fire and is the foundation for the separation of clear and turbid substances. Thus, no matter whether fire is caused by a scorched heart or by physical labor, by rich flavors and liquors, or by fire in the upper and middle burner, the five minds, mouth, or abdomen, it always must arrive at the bladder from the small intestine, descending through the clear tracts."

This quotation elaborates even more clearly on the pathomechanism by which bloody urine can result from the heart spreading heat to the small intestine.

📖 *Xuè Zhèng Lùn* ("Treatise on Blood Patterns"), "On the Pathomechanisms of the Bowels and Viscera"

"[The heart] is linked to the small intestine in an exterior-interior relationship. Heat spreading into the small intestine causes red urine."

This quotation points out that heart heat spreading downward to the small intestine decocts the urinary humors, causing red or yellow urine.

📖 *Xuè Zhèng Lùn* ("Treatise on Blood Patterns"), "Bloody Urine"

"Internal causes refer to emission of heat from the heart channel into the small intestine and emission of heat from the liver channel into the blood chamber. When the pattern manifests as strangury with constipation, cutting pain, and urinary dripping or stoppage, it is called "red strangury.""

This quotation points out that when heat spreads downward from the heart to the small intestine and the bladder fails to perform its function of transforming qì, urinary dribbling, roughness, and pain will result. It is sometimes questioned that the heart spreads heat downward to the small intestine since, from the perspective of Western medicine, pathological changes in the small intestine have no direct relationship with urination. Nonetheless, the process of heart fire spreading downward to the small intestine, resulting in red and rough urine or bloody urine, is an existing pathomechanism. It is evidenced by the large amount of discussion mentioned above, as well as by the traditional theory that the small intestine separates the clear from the turbid and governs the humors.

文献评述

《素问•痿论》说："悲哀太甚，则包络绝，包络绝则阳气内动，发则心下崩，数溲血也。"心包络为心之外卫，阳气内动，是因心火亢盛，引起尿频数、尿血，是心与小肠相合，心火下移小肠所致。

《诸病源候论•血病诸候》说："心主于血，与小肠合。若心家有热，结于小肠，故小便血也。"明确指出心经有热，可通过经脉相传，下移小肠，迫血妄行而引起尿血。

《景岳全书•杂证膜•血证》：说"溺孔之血，其来远者，出自小肠。其证则溺孔不痛，而血随溺出，或痛隐于脐腹，或热见于脏腑。盖小肠与心为表里，此丙火气化之源，清浊所由以分也。故无论焦心劳力，或厚味酒浆，而上中二焦五志口腹之火，凡从清道以降者，必皆由小肠以达膀胱也。"更清楚阐述心移热小肠可引起尿血的病机。

《血证论•脏腑病机论》说："与小肠相为表里，移热于小肠，则小便赤。"指出心热下移小肠，煎熬尿液，可使小便黄赤。

《血证论•尿血》说："内因，乃心经遗热于小肠，肝经遗热于血室。其证淋秘割痛，小便点滴不通者，呼赤淋。"指出心热下移小肠，膀胱气化失职，可致小便淋漓涩痛。有人对心移热小肠提出质疑，因为从西医的观点来看，小肠病变与排尿无直接关联。但从上述大量论证，结合小肠泌别清浊、主液的传统理论，心火下移小肠而致小便赤涩、尿血是客观存在的病机。

Summary of Upward Flaming and Downward Spreading of Heart Fire

1. Flaming Upward to the Head and Face
   Ascending to harass the face: Red eyes, redness of the whole face, sores on the face
   Ascending to harass the tongue: Sores of the mouth and tongue; erosion, swelling and pain; a red-tipped tongue; swelling of the tongue; spontaneous bleeding of the tongue; protrusion or worrying of the tongue; possibly a double tongue
2. Fire Spreading Downward to the Small Intestine
   Poor qì transformation: Red or yellow urine, hot or painful urination, stagnant, rough, and inhibited urination
   Heat damaging the blood network vessels: Bloody urine

上炎下移
上炎头面 　　上扰于面 —— 目睛红赤、满面通红、面部疮疡。 　　上扰于舌 —— 口舌生疮、糜烂肿痛，舌尖红赤、舌肿、舌衄、 　　吐舌、弄舌、重舌。 下移小肠 　　气化不行 —— 小便黄赤、尿热尿痛、滞涩不畅。 　　热伤血络 —— 尿血。

In summary, the pathomechanisms involved in exuberant yáng qì of the heart can be divided into the aspects of heat harassing the heart spirit, phlegm fire harassing the heart, heat hurrying the blood in the vessels, and upward flaming and downward spreading of heart fire. When the pathomechanism of exuberant yáng qì of the heart progresses even further, it can transform and transmute into effulgent heart and liver fire, exuberant heart and lung heat, or noninteraction of the heart and kidney.

Effulgent Heart and Liver Fire

The heart is associated with fire and the liver is associated with wood; they are interdependent on each other in a relationship of mother and child. When heart fire is exuberant, the disorder of the child affects the mother and can easily lead to stirring of liver fire. This forms the pathomechanism of effulgent heart and liver fire. In clinical practice, the symptoms of a red face and heart vexation accompanied by red eyes and irascibility are clear signs of this pattern.

Exuberant Heart and Lung Heat

The notion that "the heart spreads heat to the lungs" is found in the *Sù Wèn* ("Plain Questions") chapter, "On Qì Reversal." This occurs because the heart and lung both reside in the upper burner. Exuberance of heart yáng and internally scorching heart fire are bound to affect the lung, causing intense and exuberant lung heat. Of course, intense and exuberant heat in the lung can also cause exuberant heart fire. These factors give rise to the pathomechanism of exuberant heart and lung heat. The commonly seen combination of heart vexation and insomnia occurring simultaneously with the symptoms of cough with yellow phlegm falls into this category.

Noninteraction of Heart and Kidney

The heart is associated with fire and the kidney is associated with water. Water and fire should help each other. If there is intense internal heart fire scorching and damaging heart yīn, there will be heart yīn depletion and sapping of kidney yīn. Water and fire then fail to help each other, resulting in the pathomechanism of noninteraction of the heart and kidney. Of course, in clinical practice, a more commonly seen process involves depleted kidney yīn failing to ascend and nourish heart yīn. This causes heart fire to become hyperactive and is another pathomechanism involved in noninteraction of the heart and kidney. These patients will suffer from pathoconditions manifesting with heart vexation and insomnia, along with limp aching lumbus and knees or seminal emission.

心的阳气亢盛在病机变化上归纳起来可分为热扰心神，痰火扰心，热迫血脉，上炎下移等几个方面。心的阳气亢盛进一步发展可引起心肝火旺，心肺热盛，心肾不交等病机变化。

心肝火旺：心火肝木，母子相依，当心火亢盛时，子病及母，易于引动肝火，形成心肝火旺的病机。临床当面红心烦时，常兼目赤易怒等症即是明证。

心肺热盛：早在《素问·气厥论》就有"心移热于肺"之说，是因心肺同居上焦，心阳亢盛，心火内灼，势必波及于肺，引起肺热炽盛；当然，肺热炽盛，亦可导致心火亢盛，从而形成心肺热盛的病机。常见心烦失眠的同时，易兼咳嗽痰黄等症，便属此类。

心肾不交：心火肾水，水火既济。若心火内炽，灼伤心阴，心阴亏损，下汲肾阴，水火失济，可引起心肾不交的病机。当然临床上更为多见的是肾阴亏虚，不能上养心阴，心火偏亢而形成心肾不交的病机。这类病人，既有心烦失眠之症，又有腰膝酸软、遗精等表现。

PART TWO

Pathomechanisms of Heart Vacuity

心虚的病机

Heart Vacuity

The qì, blood, and fluids are the material foundation that maintains the normal physiologic activity of the heart. A person's normal activities invariably cause wear on the yáng qì and yīn blood of the heart. If these are not replenished periodically or if various pathogenic factors damage the heart, the resulting pathological changes tend to fall into the category of vacuity heart disease. The natural aging process, as well as long-term illness, a prolonged course of disease, and a lack of treatment or inappropriate treatment cause a progressively heavier strain on the heart function; subsequently, the detriment to the heart gradually becomes more obvious. As a consequence, the person grows more susceptible to pathomechanisms of heart vacuity.

The text *Jǐng Yuè Quán Shū* ("Jǐng-Yuè's Complete Compendium"), in the section, "Schema of Miscellaneous Patterns: Vacuity Detriment," states,: "In all cases of taxation damage and vacuity detriment, the heart is the viscus most affected, even though all five viscera have functions to govern."

The pathomechanisms of heart vacuity were first described in the *Huáng Dì Nèi Jīng* ("The Yellow Emperor's Inner Canon"). The *Sù Wèn* ("Plain Questions"), in the chapter, "On the Formation of the Five Viscera," contains the statement, "Heart vacuity is due to excessive thought and preoccupation, from which evil follows." The *Mài Jīng* ("The Pulse Canon"), in the "Chapter on Feeling the Pulse in the Front and Back of Man's Prognosis (*rén yíng*) [ST-9], Spirit Gate (*shén mén*) [HT-7], and Qì Opening [wrist pulse]," states, "Heart vacuity is characterized by a yīn and vacuous pulse at the inch-opening of the left hand, and in front of Man's Prognosis (*rén yíng*) [ST-9]; these both correspond to the hand lesser yīn channel."

Again, a quotation from the text *Shèng Jì Zǒng Lù* ("Sages' Salvation Records"), in the section on "Heart Vacuity," states, "The condition of heart vacuity appears as debilitation and scantiness of qì and blood."

More recent medical records are often compiled in separate categories for the individual viscera, including examples such as the texts *Jì Shēng Fāng* ("Formulas for Saving Lives"), *Dān Xī Shǒu Jìng* ("Dān-Xī's Hand Mirror"), *Jǐng Yuè Quán Shū* ("Jǐng-Yuè's Complete Compendium"), and the *Bǐ Huā Yī Jìng* ("Bǐ Huā Medical Mirror"). All these texts contain exclusive chapters that discuss the pathomechanisms of heart vacuity.

The pathological changes resulting from heart vacuity can be divided into the four categories of heart qì vacuity, heart yáng vacuity (including fulminant desertion of heart yáng), heart blood vacuity, and heart yīn vacuity. By their nature, vacuity of heart qì and yáng tend toward vacuity cold, while heart vacuity of blood and yīn tend toward vacuity heat.

气血津液是维持心的正常生理活动的物质基础。在人的正常生理活动中，心的阳气、阴血会受到一定的消耗，如果得不到及时补充，或由各种致病因素作用，均会造成心的物质基础和功能活动受到损害，产生不及、减弱或衰退，从而引起心病偏虚一类的病机变化。并随着生命的进程，人的衰老，或疾病日久，病程迁延，或失治误治，心的功能负担越来越重，心的损耗逐渐显着，故易引起心虚一类的病机。如《景岳全书•杂证谟•虚损》说："凡劳伤虚损，五脏各有所主，而惟心脏最多。"心虚的病机从《黄帝内经》开始就有所论述。《素问•五藏生成篇》有"思虑而心虚，故邪从之"之说。《脉经•平人迎神门气口前后脉篇》亦说："心虚，左手寸口人迎以前脉阴虚者，手少阴经也。"《圣济总录•心虚》又说："心虚之状，气血衰少。"后世许多按脏腑分类编纂的医籍，如《济生方》、《丹溪手镜》、《景岳全书》、《笔花医镜》均专篇讨论心虚的病机。归纳而言，心虚的病机变化可分为心气虚、心阳虚（包括心阳暴脱）、心血虚和心阴虚四类。其中心的气、阳虚，性质偏于虚寒；心的血、阴虚，性质偏于虚热。

Chapter Eight

Heart Qì Vacuity

Heart qì is the material foundation for the activities of the heart. It propels the blood, vitalizes the essence-spirit, and maintains activity throughout the course of one's life. The term "heart qì vacuity" was mentioned formally in the *Huáng Dì Nèi Jīng* ("The Yellow Emperor's Inner Canon"). A quotation from the *Sù Wèn* ("Plain Questions") chapter, "Treatise on Comparative [Understanding of] Exuberance and Debilitation" states, "In cases of heart qì depletion, one dreams of fighting fire and other things of a yáng nature. At the most intense times, one dreams of blazing torches." This quotation stresses the close connection between heart qì and a person's mental and emotional activities.

The *Zhū Bìng Yuán Hòu Lùn* ("The Origin and Indicators of Disease"), in "Symptoms of Heart Disease," points out specifically, "An insufficiency of heart qì results in an enlarged chest and abdomen; painful tautness between the rib-sides, lumbus, and back; fright palpitations and abstraction; lack of color in the face; rigidity in the root of the tongue; and susceptibility to worry and sorrow. These are signs of heart qì vacuity." This quotation describes how heart qì vacuity can lead to pathological changes in the heart vessels and heart spirit. Most of the later medical texts contain developments that progress from this foundation.

Many types of pathogenic factors can cause damage to the functions of the heart and lead to heart qì vacuity. Among the externally contracted six excesses, the evils of wind, heat, dampness, and cold are most likely to assail the heart. Among the internally damaging seven affects, anxiety, sorrow, thought, and preoccupation are the most likely to damage heart qì. Pathological products that are retained in the body, in particular phlegm, rheum, water, and dampness, can easily ascend counterflow and intimidate the heart, while static blood can easily obstruct the blood vessels. Heart qì may be damaged by dietary irregularities and a predilection for acrid and spicy food, for tobacco and alcohol, or for fatty, sweet, greasy or rich foods. In addition, constitutional insufficiencies, excessive taxation fatigue, physical debilitation in old age, chronic or severe illness, and in-appropriate treatment or lack of appropriate treatment can all damage heart qì. Finally, disorders from the other bowels and viscera may be transmitted to the heart.

The pathomechanisms of heart qì vacuity manifest predominantly as lack of movement in the heart vessels, heart spirit deprived of nourishment, non-constraint of heart qì, and debilitation of ancestral qì.

心气虚

心气是心的功能活动的物质基础，能推动血液，振奋精神，维持全身生命活动。早在《黄帝内经》中已正式提出"心气虚"的名称，如《素问•方盛衰论》说："心气虚，则梦救火阳物，得其时，则梦燔灼。"提出心气与人的精神情志活动有密切关系。《诸病源候论•心病候》专门指出："心气不足，则胸腹大，胁下与腰背相引痛，惊悸恍惚，少颜色，舌本强，善忧悲，是心气之虚也。"论述了心气虚可引起心脉和心神病变。以后的大多医着都是在此基础上的进一步发展。多种致病因素可导致心功能的损害而引起心的气虚。外感六淫，风、热、湿、寒之邪最易犯心；内伤七情，忧愁思虑最易损伤心气；病理产物停留，痰、饮、水、湿易上逆凌心，瘀血容易痹阻血脉；饮食不节，嗜食辛辣烟酒、肥甘厚腻，先天不足，劳倦过度，老年体弱，久病重病，失治误治，以及其它脏腑疾病的传变，均会损伤心气。心气虚的病机主要表现为心脉失运，心神失养、心气失敛和宗气衰少等几个方面。

8.1 Lack of Movement in the Heart Vessels

Heart qì is the driving force that propels the movement of blood. When heart qì is vacuous, it lacks the strength to move the blood. The resulting abnormalities affect the way in which the heart governs the blood vessels. This manifests in various pathological changes, such as an abnormal heart beat, blood vessels that are deprived of fullness, and blood stasis due to qì vacuity.

心脉失运

心气是推动血液运行的动力。心气虚，运血无力，可引起心主血脉的功能失常，表现为心动异常，血脉失充和气虚血瘀等几个方面的病机变化。

8.1.1 Abnormal Heartbeat

In heart qì vacuity, the power of the heart is weakened, the beating of the heart viscus lack strength, and the heart pumps less blood than normal. This consequently reduces the blood supply in the entire body and compels the heart to speed up and skip beats in order to compensate for the external shortage of blood. The heart rate is accelerated, causing flusteredness. The heart may also become tired, which results in patterns of palpitations.

When heart qì is vacuous, it lacks the strength to move blood. Since heart qì is unable to propel the blood and supply the body of the heart viscus itself, the heart spirit becomes deprived of nourishment and the spirit-qì becomes unsettled. This results in feelings of apprehension and uneasiness, manifesting as heart palpitations, fear and stirring, and the subjective feeling of emptiness in the heart. It should be treated by supplementing heart qì while quieting the heart spirit. For a formula, use a modified version of Heart-Nourishing Decoction (*yǎng xīn tāng*) from the *Zhèng Zhì Zhǔn Shéng* ("The Level-Line of Pattern Identification and Treatment").

Heart-Nourishing Decoction (养心汤 *yǎng xīn tāng*)

huáng qí (黄芪 Astragali Radix, astragalus)

rén shēn (人参 Ginseng Radix, ginseng)

zhì gān cǎo (炙甘草 Glycyrrhizae Radix cum Liquido Fricta, mix-fried licorice)

fú líng (茯苓 Poria, poria)

fú shén (茯神 Poria cum Pini Radice, root poria)

dāng guī (当归 Angelicae Sinensis Radix, Chinese angelica)

chuān xiōng (川芎 Chuanxiong Rhizoma, chuanxiong)

bǎi zǐ rén (柏子仁 Platycladi Semen, arborvitae seed)

suān zǎo rén (酸枣仁 Ziziphi Spinosi Semen, spiny jujube)

yuǎn zhì (远志 Polygalae Radix, polygala)

wǔ wèi zǐ (五味子 Schisandrae Fructus, schisandra)

bàn xià qū (半夏曲 Pinelliae Massa Fermentata, pinellia leaven)

心动异常

心气虚，心力减弱，心脏搏动乏力，泵血外出减少，对全身的供血自然减少，心脏被迫加快跳动，以补偿对外供血不足，心率加快，可自觉心慌、心累而见心悸不安之症；心气虚，运血无力，不能推动血液供养心体，心神失养，神气不定，志忑不宁，故心悸惕惕而动，自觉心中空虚。治宜补心气，安心神。方用《证治准绳》

<u>养心汤</u>（黄芪、人参、炙甘草、茯苓、茯神、当归、川芎、柏子仁、酸枣仁、远志、五味、半夏曲）加减。

Literature Review of Abnormal Heartbeat

📖 *Zhū Bìng Yuán Hòu Lùn* ("The Origin and Indicators of Disease"), "Symptoms of Wind Fright Palpitations"

> Wind fright palpitations are caused by a weak constitution and an insufficiency of heart qì, which allows the palace of the heart to be seized by wind. Alternatively, heart qì vacuity that arises from a rush of fear, anxiety, or worry can also cause the heart to contract wind evil. When wind evil strikes the heart, it causes fright palpitations or incessant fright, which results in palpitations at irregular intervals."

This quotation points out that the various causative factors above may damage heart qì, resulting in vacuity of heart qì, a lack of strength for the movement of blood, and a loss of nourishment for the heart spirit. This can manifest with fright, apprehension, and heart palpitations or fearful throbbing.

📖 *Zhāng Shì Yī Tōng* ("Zhang's Clear View of Medicine"), "Palpitations"

> "Palpitations below the heart are ascribed to qì vacuity or blood vacuity, either with rheum or with fire. Qì vacuity means an internal reduction of yáng qì. The area below the heart is empty and vacuous, internal stirring causes palpitations, heart qì is unsettled, and the five viscera suffer from insufficiency."

This quotation emphasizes that heart qì vacuity causes a lack of strength for propelling blood and, in compensation, an accelerated heartbeat. Thus, the heart spirit will not be calm and stable. This pathomechanism produces heart stirring and the subjective perception of emptiness and vacuity inside the heart.

文献评述

《诸病源候论•风惊悸候》说："风惊悸者，由体虚，心气不足，心之府为风邪所乘。或恐惧忧迫，令心气虚，亦受于风邪，风邪搏于心，则惊悸不安，惊不已，则悸动不定。"指出各种原因，损伤心气，心气虚弱，运血无力，心神失养，可致惊惕不安，心悸怔忡的表现。

《张氏医通•悸》亦说："心下悸有气虚血虚，属饮属火之殊。夫气虚者，是阳气内微，心下空虚，内动为悸，心气不定，五脏不足。"强调心气虚，对心血的推动无力，代偿性地引起心跳加快，神气不能平定，而致心动不安，心中自我感觉空虚的病机。

8.1.2 Blood Vessels Deprived of Fullness

The *Sù Wèn* ("Plain Questions") chapter, "Treatise on the Six Periods and Visceral Manifestation" states, "The heart is the root of life and the transmutation of the spirit. Its bloom is in the face and its fullness is in the blood vessels." This explains that heart qì propels the blood, ascends to provide luxuriance to the face, and fills and nourishes the blood vessels in the entire body.

When heart qì is vacuous or damaged, it lacks the strength to move blood to the face. The blood vessels in the face lose fullness, resulting in a pale white, pale yellow, or withered-yellow facial complexion. When blood fails to fill the lips and tongue, it results in pale lips and a pale, thin, and small tongue.

Heart qì is closely linked to the strength, speed, and rhythm of the pulse. When heart qì is vacuous, the movement of the blood lacks strength; thus, the volume of blood is reduced and the blood loses fullness. This can manifest as a pulse that is slow, fine, faint or weak. When the vessel qì is unable to flow steadily and without interruption, it will result in a bound or regularly interrupted pulse. This condition should be treated by supplementing heart qì, and by freeing and moving the blood in the vessels. For a formula, use Four Gentlemen Decoction (*sì jūn zǐ tāng*) from the *Tài Píng Huì Mín Hé Jì Jú Fāng* ("Tài-Píng Imperial Grace Pharmacy Formulas"), with the addition of astragalus and tangkui. This supplements qì and blood so that they may ascend to provide luxuriance to the face.

Four Gentlemen Decoction (四君子汤 *sì jūn zǐ tāng*)

rén shēn (人参 Ginseng Radix, ginseng)
fú líng (茯苓 Poria, poria)
bái zhú (白术 Atractylodis Macrocephalae Rhizoma, white atractylodes)
gān cǎo (甘草 Glycyrrhizae Radix, licorice)
Plus:
huáng qí (黄芪 Astragali Radix, astragalus)
dāng guī (当归 Angelicae Sinensis Radix, Chinese angelica)

Alternatively, use a modified version of Honey-Fried Licorice Decoction (*zhì gān cǎo tāng*) from the *Shāng Hán Lùn* ("On Cold Damage"), in order to supplement qì and blood and regulate the blood in the vessels.

Honey-Fried Licorice Decoction (炙甘草汤 *zhì gān cǎo tāng*) (modified)

zhì gān cǎo (炙甘草 Glycyrrhizae Radix cum Liquido Fricta, mix-fried licorice)

guì zhī (桂枝 Cinnamomi Ramulus, cinnamon twig)

rén shēn (人参 Ginseng Radix, ginseng)

shēng dì huáng (生地黄 Rehmanniae Radix Exsiccata seu Recens, dried/fresh rehmannia)

ē jiāo (阿胶 Asini Corii Colla, ass hide glue)

mài dōng (麦冬 Ophiopogonis Radix, ophiopogon)

huǒ má rén (火麻仁 Cannabis Fructus, cannabis fruit)

dà zǎo (大枣 Jujubae Fructus, jujube)

血脉失充

《素问•六节藏象论》说："心者，生之本，神之变也，其华在面，其充在血脉。"说明心气能推动血液，上荣于面，充养血脉于全身。心气虚损，无力运血于面，面部血脉失充，则为面色淡白、淡黄或萎黄；不能充盈于唇舌，则见唇舌色淡、舌体瘦小。心气与脉动的强弱和快慢、节律有密切关系。心气虚，运血无力，血少失充，可见迟脉、细脉、微脉、弱脉；脉气不相接续，则为结或代脉。治宜补养心气，通行血脉。方用《太平惠民和剂局方》四君子汤（人参、茯苓、白术、甘草）加黄芪、当归，补养气血，上荣于面；或用《伤寒论》炙甘草汤（炙甘草、桂枝、人参、生地、阿胶、麦冬、火麻仁、大枣）加减，补养气血，调整血脉。

Literature Review of Blood Vessels Deprived of Fullness

📖 *Zhū Bìng Yuán Hòu Lùn* ("The Origin and Indicators of Disease"), "Symptoms of Heart Disease"

> "When heart qì is insufficient… [it manifests as] scantiness of color."

When heart qì is vacuous, it is unable to propel qì and blood. Thus, they cannot ascend to provide luxuriance to the face; the blood network vessels in the face will be deprived of fullness, and the facial complexion will be pale white with little color.

📖 *Shèng Jì Zǒng Lù* ("Sages' Salvation Records"), "Heart Vacuity"

> "In the condition of heart vacuity, there is debility of qì, scantiness of blood, and a sallow face."

This quotation points out that when heart qì is vacuous, it is unable to propel qì and blood to ascend in order to provide luxuriance to the face. Thus, the blood vessels in the face will be deprived of nourishment; this can cause a pale white or pale yellow facial complexion.

📖 *Jǐng Yuè Quán Shū* ("Jǐng-Yuè's Complete Compendium"), "Schema of Miscellaneous Patterns, Disorders of the Face"

> "When patients have a white-colored face, it indicates qì vacuity. Alternatively, if a complexion that is both white and pale yellow is accompanied by qì insufficiency, it invariably indicates a loss of blood."

In cases of qì vacuity, the face will be white or pale yellow because heart qì is the main force that moves blood to provide luxuriance to the face. Thus, when heart qì is vacuous, it is unable to ascend to provide luxuriance to the face.

文献评述

　　《诸病源候论·心病候》说："心气不足，…少颜色。"心气虚，不能推动气血上荣于面，面部血络失充，故面色淡白而少颜色。

　　《圣济总录·心虚》说："心虚之状，气血衰少，面黄。"指出心气虚，不能推动气血上荣于面，面部血脉失养，可致面色淡白或淡黄。

　　《景岳全书·杂证谟·面病》亦说："病人面色白者气虚也，或白兼淡黄而气不足者，必失血。"在气虚中，心气是运血荣面的主要动力，故面白或淡黄，与心气虚不能上荣于面有关。

8.1.3　Blood Stasis due to Qì Vacuity

The movement of blood is dependent on the propelling action of qì to circulate incessantly. When heart qì is vacuous, it lacks the strength to move blood. Thus, the blood flow slows down and gradually stagnates. This forms the pathomechanism of blood stasis due to qì vacuity.

This concept is stated explicitly in the *Yī Lín Gǎi Cuò* ("Correction of Errors in Medical Classics") chapter, "Discussing the Fact that Tugging Wind is not Wind." It states, "Since the original qì is vacuous, it invariably lacks the ability to reach the blood in the vessels. When the blood in the vessels is deprived of qì, it invariably pauses and stops, resulting in stasis." While this quotation does not yet clearly indicate the pathomechanism of heart qì vacuity causing stasis, it is common knowledge that heart qì is the main force for propelling the blood flow and that original qì vacuity must include heart qì.

When heart qì is vacuous, it is unable to move blood through the vessels; thus, the blood vessels in the body of the heart become static. Because lack of free flow causes pain, this frequently manifests in symptoms such as pain in the heart and chest and a feeling of being pricked by needles. The location of the pain is fixed and sensitive to pressure.

If heart qì is weak and the heart and liver are both affected, there will be stagnation of liver blood, which usually manifests as swelling in the rib-sides with pain that stretches into the chest and back. As the *Zhū Bìng Yuán Hòu Lùn* ("The Origin and Indicators of Disease"), in the section on "Symptoms of Heart Disease," states, "When heart qì is insufficient, the chest and abdomen will be enlarged; pain will stretch into the area under the rib-sides and the back." This may correspond approximately to the modern diagnosis of heart failure. Here, the qì and blood of the heart and liver are static, leading to hepatosplenomegaly.

If weakness of heart qì causes qì to lose its propelling force, the flow of blood in the face is inhibited and the blood in the network vessels stagnates. This causes the facial complexion to be dark and dull or soot black. If the lips are affected by inhibited blood flow, they will become blue-green or purple; if the tongue is affected, it may become dark and dull, with stasis macules or stasis speckles. If the nails are affected by inhibited blood flow, they will become blue-green or purple. If the qì and blood stagnate in the blood vessels, one will observe a rough, bound or regularly interrupted pulse.

The treatment for blood stasis due to qì vacuity involves supplementing qì and blood while quickening blood and transforming stasis. For a formula, use Yáng-Supplementing Five-Returning Decoction (*bǔ yáng huán wǔ tāng*) from the *Yī Lín Gǎi Cuò* ("Correction of Errors in Medical Classics"), with the addition of ginseng, cinnamon twig, and honey-fried licorice.

Yáng-Supplementing Five-Returning Decoction (补阳还五汤 *bǔ yáng huán wǔ tāng*)
huáng qí (黄芪 Astragali Radix, astragalus)
dāng guī (当归 Angelicae Sinensis Radix, Chinese angelica)
chì sháo (赤芍 Paeoniae Radix Rubra, red peony)
dì lóng (地龙 Pheretima, earthworm)
chuān xiōng (川芎 Chuanxiong Rhizoma, chuanxiong)
táo rén (桃仁 Persicae Semen, peach kernel)
hóng huā (红花 Carthami Flos, carthamus)
Plus:
rén shēn (人参 Ginseng Radix, ginseng)

guì zhī (桂枝 Cinnamomi Ramulus, cinnamon twig)
zhì gān cǎo (炙甘草 Glycyrrhizae Radix cum Liquido Fricta,
mix-fried licorice)

气虚血瘀

血之运行，有赖于气之推动，方能循环不息。心气虚，运血无力，血行迟缓，渐至停滞，引起气虚血瘀之病机。正如《医林改错•论抽风不是风》所云："元气既虚，必不能达于血管，血管无气，必停留而瘀。"此处虽未明确提出心气虚致瘀的病机，但众所周知，心气是推动血行的主要动力，元气虚必然包括心气在内。心气虚，不能鼓动心脉，心体血脉瘀阻，不通则痛，故常见心胸疼痛、有针刺感、痛处固定、不喜压按等表现。若心气虚弱，心肝同病，导致肝血瘀滞，常见胁肋肿大，胸背引痛的表现。如《诸病源候论•心病候》说："心气不足，则胸腹大，胁下与背相引痛。"相当于现代心力衰竭时，心肝气血瘀滞而引起肝脾肿大的表现。若心气虚弱，气失推动，面部血脉不畅，血络瘀滞，则为面色晦暗或黧黑；唇舌血络不畅，则为唇舌青紫，或舌质晦暗，有瘀斑、瘀点；爪甲血络不行，则为爪甲青紫。血脉气血阻滞，则见涩脉、结脉或代脉。治宜补养心气，活血化瘀。方选《医林改错》补阳还五汤（黄芪、当归、赤芍、地龙、川芎、桃仁、红花）加人参、桂枝、炙甘草进行调治。

Literature Review of Blood Stasis due to Qì Vacuity

📖 *Zhū Bìng Yuán Hòu Lùn* ("The Origin and Indicators of Disease"),
"Symptoms of Throat, Heart, and Chest Disorders, "Symptoms of
Heart Impediment"

"Excessive thought, preoccupation, and vexation damage the heart.
When the heart is vacuous, evil can exploit it. When the evil accumulates
and does not go, the person periodically sustains damage from food or
drink, causing depression in the heart as if in a state of fullness, with
seething and pain. This is the condition called heart impediment."

Moreover, the commentary points out in greater detail:

"Excessive thought, preoccupation, vexation, and taxation can damage
heart qì. This causes heart qì vacuity detriment, which results in binding
depression affecting the heart. This presents with oppression and dull
pain, and is known as a heart impediment disorder."

This quotation points out that thought and preoccupation can damage the
heart. When heart qì is weak, it is unable to propel the movement of blood;
this results in heart vessel obstruction and pain in the heart and chest.

📖 *Líng Shū* ("The Magic Pivot"), "Chapter on the Channels and Vessels"

> "Qì expiry in the hand lesser yīn channel causes stoppage in the vessels. When there is stoppage in the vessels, blood does not flow. When blood does not flow, the complexion will be lusterless. If the face becomes black like lacquered kindling, the blood has already died."

Qì expiry in the hand lesser yīn channel refers to heart qì debility; the heart loses its propelling strength, resulting in blood stasis. The color of the static blood manifests externally as a somber facial complexion.

文献评述

《诸病源候论校释•咽喉心胸病候•心痹候》说："思虑烦多则损心，心虚故邪乘之，邪积而不去，则时害饮食，心里愊愊如满，蕴蕴而痛，是谓心痹。"并在注释中明确指出："思虑烦劳过多，能损伤心气，心气虚损，…心郁结而闷，隐隐作痛，这就称为心痹病。"指出思虑伤心，心气虚弱，不能推动血行，而致心脉痹阻，心胸疼痛。

《灵枢•经脉篇》曰："手少阴气绝，则脉不通，脉不通，则血不流，血不流则发色不泽，故面黑如漆柴者，血先死。"手少阴气绝，就是心气虚衰，失于推动，故致血瘀，瘀血之色外现，故面色晦暗。

Summary of Lack of Movement in the Heart Vessels

1. Abnormal Heartbeat
   Heart palpitations, fear, and emptiness in the heart
2. Blood Vessels Deprived of Nourishment
   Lack of luster in the face and tongue
   > Pale white, pale yellow or withered-yellow facial complexion
   > Pale lips and tongue, thin and small tongue body

   Irregular heart rate
   > *Loss of fullness in the blood vessels*: a pulse that is slow, fine, faint or weak
   > *Discontinuity of vessel qì*: the pulse is bound or intermittent
3. Blood Stasis due to Qì Vacuity
   Blood stasis in the heart vessels: heart and chest pain that feels like the stabbing of a needle; the pain is at a fixed location and is sensitive to pressure
   Blood stasis in the heart and liver: swelling and enlargement of the rib-sides with pain that stretches to the chest and back
   Inhibited blood flow in the vessels
   > *Facial complexion*: soot black or somber
   > *Lips and tongue*: dark tongue body, presence of stasis macules or stasis speckles

Nails: blue-green or purple
Pulse: rough, bound, or intermittent

心脉失运

心动异常
    心悸、惕惕不安、心中空虚。
血脉失养
    面舌失华
        面色淡白、淡黄萎黄
        唇舌色淡、舌体瘦小
    心律失调
        血脉失充 —— 迟、细、微、弱。
        脉气不续 —— 结、代。
气虚血瘀
    心脉血瘀 —— 心胸疼痛、针刺感、痛处固定、不喜压。
    心肝血瘀 —— 胁肋肿大，胸背引痛。
    血脉不畅
        面色 —— 黧黑、晦暗。
        唇舌 —— 舌质晦暗，有瘀斑、瘀点。
        爪甲 —— 青紫。
        脉搏 —— 涩、结、代

8.2   Heart Spirit Deprived of Nourishment

Heart qì sustains mental activity. Heart qì must be abundant if the heart is to receive stimuli from the environment, react correspondingly, and maintain mental activity, thought, and consciousness. If heart qì is damaged, the heart spirit is deprived of nourishment; this can easily affect its ability to perform normal mental activities. This process is involved in many pathomechanisms associated with mental irregularities.

The chapter "Explaining Internal Damage" in the *Yī Lǐ Zhēn Chuán* ("True Transmission of Medical Principles") states: "All cases associated with internal damage are attributable first to a despoliation of heart qì; the spirit fails to be governed, so it is unable to maintain its hold over the hundred offices. Thus, various pathoconditions arise."

The changes in the heart spirit caused by heart qì vacuity detriment can be divided into the categories of insufficiency of spirit qì, mental derangement, and dissipation and desertion of the heart spirit.

心神失养

心气是维持人的精神活动的动力条件。心气旺盛，才能接受外界各种刺激，作出应答反应，主持精神思维意识活动。若心气损伤，心神失养，就会失却正常的精神活动，引起多种精神失调的病机变化。正如《医理真传·内伤说》所云："凡属内伤者，皆心气先夺，神无所主，不能镇定百官，诸症于是蜂起矣。"心气虚损引起心神变化可分为神气不足，精神错乱和心神散脱等几个方面。

8.2.1   Insufficiency of Spirit Qì

Spirit qì supports the normal activities of the heart spirit. It allows one's energy to flow copiously and allows the mind to be concentrated and attentive. It allows one's thinking to leap and bound, giving one sharp and sensitive responses and general intelligence and wisdom. Thus, an individual may "respond to their environment according to the circumstances, through a thousand changes and myriad transformations" (*Lèi Jīng* ("The Classified Canon"), "Categories of Visceral Manifestation").

If the heart qì is depleted, it becomes unable to provide the material foundation for the activities of the heart spirit. The ability of the heart to govern the spirit-mind may then become reduced or weakened. As a result, the heart spirit becomes unable to govern itself and the spirit qì becomes disquieted. This can cause a subjective feeling of emptiness in the heart and anxiety. Alternatively, the essence-spirit can become timid and weak and courage may be reduced; this manifests as timidity in the heart, fearfulness and susceptibility to fright, and damaging amounts of anxiety, worry, and sorrow.

Spirit qì debility may reach the point where it is unable to support the ordinary activities of the mind, thoughts, and consciousness. The essence-spirit will be exhausted, causing scattered thoughts, difficult concentration, and delayed and dull responses. If the heart spirit is deprived of nourishment, the spirit-mind will not be calm; this manifests as superficial and easily disturbed sleep, sleeplessness and profuse dreaming or constant sleepiness and spontaneous waking from sound sleep. This should be treated by supplementing heart qì while quieting the spirit and settling fright. For a formula, use Spirit-Quieting Mind-Stabilizing Pill (*ān shén dìng zhì wán*) from the *Yī Xué Xīn Wù* ("Medical Insights"), combined with Poria Heart-Supplementing Decoction (*fú líng bǔ xīn tāng*) from the *Qiān Jīn Yào Fāng* ("A Thousand Gold Pieces Prescriptions").

Spirit-Quieting Mind-Stabilizing Pill (安神定志丸 *ān shén dìng zhì wán*)

rén shēn (人参 Ginseng Radix, ginseng)
fú líng (茯苓 Poria, poria)

fú shén (茯神 Poria cum Pini Radice, root poria)
yuǎn zhì (远志 Polygalae Radix, polygala)
shí chāng pú (石菖蒲 Acori Tatarinowii Rhizoma, acorus)
lóng chǐ (龙齿 Mastodi Dentis Fossilia, dragon tooth)

Poria Heart-Supplementing Decoction (补心汤 *fú líng bǔ xīn tāng*)

fú líng (茯苓 Poria, poria)
guì xīn (桂心 Cinnamomi Cortex Rasus, shaved cinnamon bark)
rén shēn (人参 Ginseng Radix, ginseng)
zǐ shí yīng (紫石英 Fluoritum, fluorite)
mài dōng (麦冬 Ophiopogonis Radix, ophiopogon)
chì xiǎo dòu (赤小豆 Phaseoli Semen, rice bean)
dà zǎo (大枣 Jujubae Fructus, jujube)

In the majority of cases of heart qì vacuity, qì vacuity and fatigue of the spirit tend to manifest in the symptoms of encumbrance, fatigue, and somnolence. However, it is also possible that debility of heart qì may result in insomnia and profuse dreaming. This occurs because the heart spirit is deprived of nourishment by heart qì, preventing it from sustaining normal mental activities and causing it to fail to keep the spirit to its abode. If one is unaware of this pathomechanism and only knows that sleeplessness results from an insufficiency of yīn-blood in the heart or an exuberance of heart fire, this can often lead to incorrect pattern identification.

神气不足

心气能维持正常的心神活动，使人精力充沛，精神集中，思维活跃，反应灵敏，具有聪明智慧，能"随机应境，千变万化"（《类经•藏象类》）。若心气亏损，不能提供心神活动的物质基础，心主神志的功能就会减弱，心神不能自主，神气不安，则会自觉心中空虚、惶惶不安；或精神怯弱，胆量变小，而见心中胆怯、恐惧易惊、忧愁悲伤；或神气衰减，不能维持正常的精神、思维、意识活动，则精神疲乏不振、思想分散不易集中、思维反应迟钝；或因心神失养，神志不得安宁，而见睡眠表浅易惊、不寐多梦、或时时欲睡、睡中自醒等症。治宜补养心气，安神镇惊。方用《医学心悟》安神定志丸《人参、茯苓、茯神、远志、石菖蒲、龙齿》合《千金要方》补心茯苓汤（茯苓、桂心、人参、紫石英、麦冬、赤小豆、大枣）。大多数心气虚者，多因气虚神疲而易表现为困倦嗜睡的症状，但确有因心气虚衰，心神缺乏心气的供养，不能主持正常的精神活动，神不守舍，而致失眠多梦。如果不识此类病机，只知心的阴血不足或心火亢盛才能引起失眠，常会导致辨证失误。

Literature Review of Insufficiency of Spirit Qì

📖 *Zhōng Zàng Jīng* ("Central Treasury Canon"), "On Methods for [Distinguishing Between] Vacuity and Repletion, Cold and Heat, Life and Death, and Smoothness and Counterflow in the Heart Viscus"

"Vacuity results in fear and susceptibility to fright, anxiety, and unhappiness."

This quotation points out that the heart spirit is deprived of nourishment in cases of heart vacuity. This can cause irregularities in the heart's ability to govern the mind, thoughts, and consciousness, resulting in many types of pathomechanisms that relate to mental and emotional irregularities, such as timidity in the heart or fear and susceptibility to fright.

📖 *Zhèng Zhì Zhǔn Shéng* ("The Level-Line of Pattern Identification and Treatment"), "Palpitations"

"There are no more than two causes of heart palpitations, vacuity and rheum. As for qì vacuity, it is due to an internal vacuity of yáng qì; there is emptiness below the heart and internal stirring of fire qì, resulting in palpitations."

This quotation points out that heart qì vacuity presents with insufficiency in the heart and disquieted spirit qì, which causes heart palpitations.

📖 *Zhèng Zhì Huì Bǔ* ("A Supplement to Patterns and Treatment"), "Heart Palpitations and Fearful Throbbing"

"Causes include: hearing a loud noise, seeing strange sights, encountering danger and facing peril, losing one's mind after a traumatic experience, or great fright and great fear. The heart becomes defiant, leading to heart vacuity and collecting rheum. This causes a state of apprehensiveness. In severe cases, it leads to heart throbbing verging on reversal and is identifiable by a slippery pulse."

This quotation points out that damage to the heart from fear weakens heart qì. In conjunction with a simultaneous arrival of phlegm-rheum, this can cause irregularities of the heart spirit, resulting in fear, stirring, and disquietude in the heart.

📖 *Jīn Guì Yào Lüè* ("Essential Prescriptions of the Golden Coffer"), "Wind-Cold Accumulating and Gathering in the Five Viscera"

"In cases when evil crying disquiets the ethereal and corporeal souls, blood and qì are scant. Cases of scant blood and qì are ascribed to the heart. When heart qì is vacuous, the person has fear, closed eyes and desire for sleep, dreams of travels afar, and has a scattered and dissipated essence-spirit and frenetic movement of the ethereal and corporeal souls."

When heart qì is vacuous, qì and blood fail to nourish the spirit and the spirit fails to keep to its abode. This causes sleeplessness and profuse dreaming.

📖 *Zhèng Yīn Mài Zhì* ("Pathoconditions: Causes, Pulses, and Treatments"), "Sleeplessness due to Heart Qì Vacuity"

"Heart qì vacuity sleeplessness is caused by a constitutional shortage of true yáng that prevents wood from engendering fire, causing heart qì vacuity. Consequently, the heart lacks the power to govern, the heart spirit fails to keep to its abode, and the pathocondition of unquiet sleep arises."

Again, it states:

"The pathocondition of heart qì vacuity sleeplessness presents with periodic efflux of stool and urine, diffuse eyes and a clear spirit, qì timidity, fatigue and lassitude, a shivering heart and a cold gallbladder, frequent desire to sleep, spontaneous awakening from sleep, preference for heat, and aversion to cold."

This quotation clearly points out that the pathomechanism of heart qì vacuity can cause a disquieted heart spirit, insomnia, and susceptibility to fright.

文献评述

《中藏经•论心脏虚实寒热生死逆顺之法》曰："虚则恐惧多惊，忧思不乐。"指出心虚，心神失养，可使心主精神、思维、意识的功能失调，引起心中胆怯，恐惧易惊等多种精神、情志失调的病机。

《证治准绳•悸》说："心悸之由，不越二种：一者虚也，二者饮也。气虚者，由阳气内虚，心下空虚，火气内动而为悸也。"指出心气虚，心中不足，神气不宁，可致心悸。

《证治汇补•心悸怔忡》说："或耳闻大声，目见异物，遇险临危，触事丧志，大惊大恐，心为之忤，以致心虚停痰，使人有惕惕之状，甚则心跳欲厥，其脉滑者是也。"指出惊恐伤心，心气虚弱，兼夹痰饮，可使人心神失调，引起心中惊动不安。

《金匮要略•五脏风寒积聚篇》曰："邪哭使魂魄不安者，血气少也。血气少者属于心，心气虚者，其人则畏，合目欲眠，梦远行而精神离散，魂魄妄行。"心气虚，气血失于养神，神不守舍，故失眠多梦。

《症因脉治•心气虚不得卧》说："心气虚不得卧之因，真阳素乏，木不生火，心气虚则心无主威，心神失守，而夜卧不安之症作矣。"又说："心气虚不得卧之症，二便时滑，目漫神清，气怯倦

怠，心战胆寒，时时欲睡，睡中自醒，喜热恶冷，此心气虚不得卧
之症也。"明确指出心气虚的病机可使人心神不安而失眠易惊。

8.2.2   Mental Derangement

The *Sù Wèn* ("Plain Questions") chapter, "Treatise of the Arcane Book of
the Orchid Chamber of the Spirit Tower" states, "The heart holds the office of monarch, whence the spirit light emanates." The heart is the place
where the essence-spirit abides, and one's mental activities are closely
connected with heart qì.

When heart qì is exuberant and reins in the spirit light, then the spirit,
essence, and mind are clear, the head and brain have bright essence, and
the essence-spirit is not deranged. If the heart qì is depleted, the heart is
unable to govern the activities of the mind. When the spirit light is ungoverned, mental abnormalities may result. Alternatively, the heart spirit
may be harassed when there is insufficiency of heart qì with concurrent
phlegm-turbidity obstructing the orifices.

All the above circumstances can result in pathoconditions of mental
derangement, manifesting with taciturnity, muttering to oneself, deranged
speech, bouts of crying and laughing, inability to differentiate between
strangers and friends, and mental abstraction or feeble-mindedness.

When the indications for the formula Heart-Supplementing Decoction
(*bǔ xīn tāng*) are discussed in the *Shèng Jì Zǒng Lù* ("Sages' Salvation Records"), in the chapter "Heart Gate," it points out that it can be used to "treat
insufficiency of heart qì, possibly with joy, sorrow, rage, or anger…or topsy-
turvy speech." Indirectly, this quotation demonstrates that heart qì vacuity is
involved in the pathomechanisms of mental abnormalities. This condition
should be treated by supplementing heart qì and quieting the essence-spirit.
For a formula, use Heart-Assisting Stomach-Calming Decoction (*zhù xīn
píng wèi tāng*) from the *Biàn Zhèng Lù* ("Record of Pattern Identification").
This formula assists stomach qì in order to engender heart qì; it assists heart
fire and calms stomach fire to treat the irregularities of the essence-spirit.

Heart-Assisting Stomach-Calming Decoction
(助心平胃汤 *zhù xīn píng wèi tāng*)

rén shēn (人参 Ginseng Radix, ginseng)
fú shén (茯神 Poria cum Pini Radice, root poria)
bèi mǔ (贝母 Fritillariae Bulbus, fritillaria)
shén qū (神曲 Massa Medicata Fermentata, medicated leaven)
ròu guì (肉桂 Cinnamomi Cortex, cinnamon bark)
jú huā (菊花 Chrysanthemi Flos, chrysanthemum)
shí chāng pú (石菖蒲 Acori Tatarinowii Rhizoma, acorus)

suān zǎo rén (酸枣仁 Ziziphi Spinosi Semen, spiny jujube)
gān cǎo (甘草 Glycyrrhizae Radix, licorice)

For treatment, one may also choose Poria Pill (*fú líng wán*) from the *Běn Shì Fāng* (also called *Pǔ Jì Běn Shì Fāng*, "Effective Remedies for Universal Relief"). This formula nourishes the heart and quiets the heart spirit while expelling phlegm-turbidity and opening the orifices of the heart.

Poria Pill (茯苓丸 *fú líng wán*)

rén shēn (人参 Ginseng Radix, ginseng)
yuǎn zhì (远志 Polygalae Radix, polygala)
fú líng (茯苓 Poria, poria)
fú shén (茯神 Poria cum Pini Radice, root poria)
shí chāng pú (石菖蒲 Acori Tatarinowii Rhizoma, acorus)
zhū shā (朱砂 Cinnabaris, cinnabar)
tiě fěn (铁粉 Ferri Pulvis, iron powder)
bàn xià qū (半夏曲 Pinelliae Massa Fermentata, pinellia leaven)
dǎn xīng (胆星 Arisaema cum Bile, bile arisaema)

精神错乱

"心为君主之官，神明出焉"（《素问•灵兰秘典》）。心为精神之所舍，人的精神活动与心气密切相关。心气充盛，驾驭神明则神精志朗，头脑精明，精神不乱。若心气亏损，不能主司精神活动，神明无主，可致精神失常；或心气不足，兼有痰浊阻窍，扰乱心神，均可引起沉默寡言、喃喃自语、言语错乱、时哭时笑、不识亲疏、精神恍惚或痴呆等精神错乱之症。如《圣济总录•心藏门》论述补心汤主治时，指出可用于"治心气不足，或喜或悲，或嗔或怒，…言语颠倒。"间接论证心气虚可引起精神失常的病机。治宜补心气、安精神。方用《辨证录》助心平胃汤（人参、茯神、贝母、神曲、肉桂、菊花、石菖蒲、生枣仁、甘草）助胃气以生心气，助心火而平胃火以治精神失常。也可选用《本事方》茯苓丸（人参、远志、茯苓、茯神、石菖蒲、辰砂、真铁粉、半夏曲、胆南星）养心气、安心神、祛痰浊，开心窍。

Literature Review of Mental Derangement

📖 *Zá Bìng Yuán Liú Xī Zhú* ("Incisive Light on the Source of Miscellaneous Disease"), "The Source of Mania and Withdrawal"

"Withdrawal is caused by heart qì vacuity and the presence of heat."

Again, it states:

"The disease of withdrawal may be caused by insufficiency of heart qì causing the spirit to fail to keep to its abode."

These quotations point out that the manifestations of mental abnormalities such as withdrawal disease can be caused by heart qì weakness. The heart spirit is deprived of nourishment and fails to govern the spirit-mind.

📖 *Biàn Zhèng Lù* ("Record of Pattern Identification"), "Entry on Withdrawal and Epilepsy"

"There are people with a chronic and untreatable predisposition for frequent attacks of withdrawal. [During attacks,] they mutter incessantly, occasionally lose consciousness, at one moment shout curses, and at the next moment sing songs, and vomit phlegm of a consistency like the drool-like mucus of slugs. When one administers phlegm-dispersing drool-transforming medicinals in such cases, they are often ineffective... Withdrawal disorders may be eliminated if the treatment utilizes Heart-Assisting Stomach-Calming Decoction... This formula supplements stomach qì to engender heart qì."

The quotation explains that heart qì vacuity causes the heart spirit to be deprived of nourishment. Thus, it fails to govern the spirit-mind. This may manifest in many types of mental derangement.

文献评述

《杂病源流犀烛•癫狂源流》说："癫由心气虚，有热。"又说："而癫之病，...有因心气不足，神不守舍者。"指出癫病等精神失常的表现，可由心气虚弱，心神失养，神志无主引起。

《辨证录•癫痫门》说："人有素常发癫，久而不效，口中喃喃不已，时时忽忽不知，时而叫骂，时而歌唱，吐痰如蜒蚰之涎。然以消痰、化涎之药与之，多不效。"在治疗时采用"补胃气以生心气"的助心平胃汤而癫病得除。说明心气虚，心神失养，神志无主，可引起多种精神错乱的表现。

8.2.3   Dissipation and Desertion of the Heart Spirit

The spirit is the external manifestation of the vital activities of the human body. When the spirit is preserved, there is life, when the spirit collapses, there is death. The material foundation of the spirit comes from qì and blood. The heart governs the blood and therefore also governs the spirit-mind.

If heart qì is vacuous, it is unable to propel the blood to nourish the heart spirit, so the heart spirit will be deprived of nourishment. In mild cases, there will be a disquieted spirit-mind. This manifests in pathoconditions of a clouded head and flowery vision, fright palpitations, forgetfulness, insomnia, and profuse dreaming.

In severe cases, heart qì will be greatly damaged; the heart spirit will become dissipated and chaotic, and the spirit will fail to keep within and will desert outward. This manifests as an unclear spirit-mind, clouded consciousness, coma or unconsciousness, possibly with a faint low voice and repetitive or disjointed speech. If the illness progresses, the person's life will be in grave danger, eventually ending in death. This condition should be treated by supplementing the heart, nourishing qì, and stemming desertion. For a formula, choose Pure Ginseng Decoction (*dú shēn tāng*) from the *Shí Yào Shén Shū* ("The Divine Text of Ten Medicinals").

Pure Ginseng Decoction (独参汤 *dú shēn tāng*)

rén shēn (人参 Ginseng Radix, ginseng)

心神散脱

神是人体生命活动的外在表现，神存则生，神亡则死。神的物质基础源于气血。心主血，故主神志。如果心气虚弱，不能推动血液奉养心神，心神失养，轻则神志不宁，出现头昏眼花、惊悸健忘、失眠多梦诸症。 重则心气大伤，心神散乱，神不内守而外脱，表现为神志不清、意识模糊、昏迷不省人事、伴见语声低微、语言重复、不相接续等表现，进而生命垂危而死亡。治宜补心养气固脱，方选《十药神书》独参汤（人参）。

Literature Review of Dissipation and Desertion of the Heart Spirit

📖 *Líng Shū* ("The Magic Pivot"), "Chapter on Visiting Evil"

> "The heart is the great governor of the five viscera and six bowels, as well as the abode of the essence-spirit. It stores firmly and securely and cannot contain evils. If they are contained within, the heart is damaged. When the heart is damaged, the spirit leaves. When the spirit leaves, the person dies."

The heart governs the spirit-mind. Although the damage sustained by the heart can be divided into qì, blood, yīn, and yáng, it invariably includes heart qì. This quotation explains that great damage to the heart qì causes the heart spirit to become dissipated and chaotic; this is a critical condition.

📖 *Sù Wèn* ("Plain Questions"), "Treatise on the Essential Subtleties of the Pulse"

> "Faint and repetitive speech is a sign of despoliated qì."

Based on the expression, "speech constitutes the sound of the heart," this quotation explains that despoliated qì is naturally caused by great damage to the heart qì; the heart spirit fails to be governed, manifesting in changes in the voice.

📖 *Jǐng Yuè Quán Shū* ("Jǐng-Yuè's Complete Compendium"), "Canon of Cold Damage: Delirious Speech and Muttering"

"Muttering is due to vacuity; vacuity refers to vacuity of the spirit. If cold damage causes the original spirit to fail to keep to its abode, [the spirit] is overwhelmed by evil and the spirit-mind becomes dazed and deranged. This is a condition of vacuity evil.

In disorders of vacuity evil, the voice is low, breathing is short, the pulse is without strength, and the complexion is withered and sallow. Signs of this condition include speaking to oneself, muttering in incomplete sentences, seeing apparitions of ghosts, incessantly experiencing fear and fright, and being non-responsive to inquiry or answering incomprehensibly. In this disease…the presence of burning thoughts or restrained depression exhausts heart qì."

This quotation explains that great damage to heart qì can result in the critical, severe pathomechanism of dissipation and desertion of the heart spirit.

文献评述

　　《灵枢•邪客篇》说："心者五脏六腑之大主也，精神之所舍也，其藏坚固，邪弗能容。容之则心伤，心伤则神去，神去则死矣。"心主神志，心受损伤虽然有气血阴阳之分，但必然包括心气，说明心气大伤，可使心神散乱，生命垂危。

　　《素问•脉要精微论》亦说："言而微，终日乃复言者，此夺气也"，由于"言为心声"，说明夺气自然是由心气大伤，心神失主而引起的语声变化。

　　《景岳全书•伤寒典•谵语郑声》说："郑声为虚，虚者神虚也，如伤寒元神失守，为邪所乘，神志昏沉而错乱不正者，此虚邪也。虚邪为病，其声必低，其气必短，其脉必无力，其色必萎悴，凡其自言自语，喃喃不全，或见鬼怪，或惊恐不休，或问之不应，答之不知之类皆是也。此之为病，…有焦思抑郁，竭尽心气而然者。"充分说明，心气大伤，可引起心神散脱等危重病机。

Summary of Heart Spirit Deprived of Nourishment

1. **Heart Spirit Insufficiency**
   Ungoverned heart spirit: Emptiness in the heart and fear

> *Timidity of the essence-spirit*: Lack of courage in the heart; fear, apprehension, and susceptibility to fright; damage from anxiety and sorrow
> *Debility of spirit qì*: Devitalized essence-spirit, scattered thinking, delayed and dull reactions
> *Disquieted spirit-mind*: Susceptibility to fright during sleep, sleeplessness and profuse dreaming, easy arousal from sleep

2. Mental Derangement

   Taciturnity, muttering to oneself, deranged speech, bouts of crying and laughing, inability to differentiate between strangers and friends, mental abstraction, or feeble-mindedness

3. Dissipation and Desertion of the Heart Spirit

   > *Disquieted spirit-qì*: Clouded head and flowery vision, fright palpitations and forgetfulness, insomnia, and profuse dreaming
   > *Dissipated and chaotic heart spirit*: Unclear spirit-mind, clouded consciousness, coma, faint low voice, repetitive or disjointed speech

心神失养
神气不足 　心神无主 —— 心中空虚、惶惶不安。 　精神怯弱 —— 心中胆怯、恐惧易惊、忧愁悲伤。 　神气衰减 —— 精神不振、思想分散、反应迟钝。 　神志不宁 —— 睡眠易惊、不寐多梦、睡眠易醒。 精神错乱 　沉默寡言、喃喃自语、言语错乱、时哭时笑、不识亲疏、精神恍惚或痴呆。 心神散脱 　神气不宁 —— 头昏眼花、惊悸健忘、失眠多梦。 　心神散乱 —— 神志不清、意识模糊、昏迷不醒、语声低微、语言重复、不相接续。

8.3 Non-Constraint of Heart Qi

The heart governs the blood vessels. The function of heart qì is not limited to propelling the movement of blood; the heart also secures and contains the blood. The fluids in the blood can permeate into the space between the tissues and then emerge from the muscles, interstices, skin, and hair as sweat. Thus, it is said that sweat is the humor of the heart.

When heart qì is debilitated, it is unable to constrain. Thus, its ability to secure and contain the blood is weakened. Moreover, it is unable to secure and contain sweat, which can result in spontaneous and incessant sweating.

Since movement wears qì, heart qì is further depleted after physical activity and its strength for securing and containing perspiration is further reduced. Therefore, perspiration is particularly strong after physical activity.

When heart qì is vacuous and unable to constrain the heart spirit, the heart spirit floats astray and the essence-spirit becomes scattered and chaotic. This manifests in heart palpitations, susceptibility to fright, sleeplessness, and forgetfulness. It should be treated by supplementing heart qì while astringing the heart spirit. For a formula, use Pulse-Engendering Powder (*shēng mài sǎn*) from the *Nèi Wài Shāng Biàn Huò Lùn* ("Clarification of Perplexities about Internal and External Damage"), with the addition of astragalus, dragon bone, and oyster shell.

Pulse-Engendering Powder (生脉散 *shēng mài sǎn*)
rén shēn (人参 Ginseng Radix, ginseng) *mài dōng* (麦冬 Ophiopogonis Radix, ophiopogon) *wǔ wèi zǐ* (五味子 Schisandrae Fructus, schisandra) Plus: *huáng qí* (黄芪 Astragali Radix, astragalus) *lóng gǔ* (龙骨 Mastodi Ossis Fossilia, dragon bone) *mǔ lì* (牡蛎 Ostreae Concha, oyster shell)

心气失敛

心主血脉，心气不仅有推动血液运行的作用，同时还对血液有固摄作用。血中的津液，可渗入组织间隙，再从肌腠皮毛而出，变成汗液，故有汗为心液之说。心气虚衰，不能收敛，对血液固摄功能减弱，也就不能固摄汗液，可引起自汗不止；动则耗气，活动后，心气更虚，对汗的固摄力量更差，故活动后汗出尤甚。心气虚，不能收敛心神，可致心神浮越，精神散乱，表现为心悸易惊，失眠健忘。治宜补养心气，收敛心神。方用《内外伤辨惑论》生脉散（人参、麦冬、五味子）加黄芪、龙骨、牡蛎。

Summary of Non-Constraint of Heart Qì

1. Failure to Constrain Sweat
   Spontaneous and incessant sweating, particularly after physical activity
2. Failure to Constrain the Heart Spirit
   Heart palpitations and susceptibility to fright, sleeplessness and forgetfulness

心气失敛
汗液失敛 —— 自汗不止，活动尤甚。
心神失敛 —— 心悸易惊，失眠健忘。

8.4 Ancestral Qì Debility

Heart qì is the primary force that propels the movement of blood, but lung qì assists the heart in moving blood. When the heart qì is vacuous, the movement of blood lacks strength; this invariably increases the burden of the lung qì. If this becomes a chronic condition, lung qì also becomes vacuous and ancestral qì becomes debilitated and scant.

When the function of the lung is weakened, breathing is shallow and there is shortness of breath. Faint and weak exhalations and inhalations result in a shortage of qì. The movement of qì becomes inhibited; it stops and stagnates in the chest and causes chest oppression. Therefore, insufficiency of heart qì invariably leads to vacuity of lung qì and debility of ancestral qì. This manifests in pathoconditions such as chest oppression with shortage of qì, shortness of breath and discontinuity of the breath, or hasty rapid breathing with an inability to lie flat.

Ancestral qì passes through the heart vessels to move the blood. When heart qì is vacuous and unable to constrain ancestral qì, ancestral qì is discharged to the outer body. This manifests in the apex of the heart beating so strongly that it is visible through the clothing. This condition should be treated by supplementing qì and boosting the origin. For a formula, use Origin-Preserving Decoction (*bǎo yuán tāng*) from the *Shí Fāng Gē Kuò* ("Popular Remedies in Verse").

Origin-Preserving Decoction (保元汤 *bǎo yuán tāng*)
rén shēn (人参 Ginseng Radix, ginseng)
huáng qí (黄芪 Astragali Radix, astragalus)
ròu guì (肉桂 Cinnamomi Cortex, cinnamon bark)
shēng jiāng (生姜 Zingiberis Rhizoma Recens, fresh ginger)
gān cǎo (甘草 Glycyrrhizae Radix, licorice)

宗气衰少

心气是推动血液运行的主要动力，肺气有助心行血的作用。心气虚弱，运血无力，必然增加肺气的负担，久之肺气亦虚，宗气衰少，肺功能减弱，呼吸表浅而气短；吐纳微弱而少气；气行不畅停滞胸中而胸闷。故心气不足者，势必引起肺气虚弱，宗气衰少，可见胸闷少气、气短不续、或呼吸急促、不能平卧等症。宗气贯心脉而行血，心气虚，不能收敛宗气，宗气外泄，可见心尖搏动应衣。
治宜补心益元。方用《时方歌括》<u>保元汤</u>（人参、黄芪、肉桂、生
姜、甘草。）

Literature Review of Ancestral Qi Debility

📖 *Líng Shū* ("The Magic Pivot"), "Chapter on Oral Inquiry"

> "When heart qì is tense, the airways are constrained. Constraint is inhibiting, so [the patient] sighs in order to stretch out."

This quotation points out that heart qì can influence lung qì. This leads to inhibition of the airways, chest oppression, and shortness of breath.

📖 *Zhū Bìng Yuán Hòu Lùn* ("The Origin and Indicators of Disease"), "Symptoms of a Lack of Qì"

> "People suffering from extreme vacuity have reduced and worn construction and defense, vacuous bowels and viscera, and insufficient movement of qì. Thus, their breathing is characterized by shortness of breath."

The heart governs construction and defense. When construction and defense are decreased and worn, it is mostly related to heart qì debility. When this involves ancestral qì, it causes weakness of qì and incomplete exhalation and inhalation; thus, the frequency of respiration is accelerated and there is shortness of breath.

📖 *Zhū Bìng Yuán Hòu Lùn* ("The Origin and Indicators of Disease"), "Symptoms of Qì Shortage"

> "This condition is caused by an insufficiency of visceral qì. The lung governs qì and facilitates breathing. When visceral qì is insufficient, it results in faint weak breathing and shortage of qì."

In this quotation, visceral qì refers to the qì of the five viscera in general. Thus, this quotation also includes heart qì insufficiency, which influences the lung and leads to shortness of breath and shortage of qì.

文献评述

　　《灵枢•口问篇》说："心气急则气道约，约则不利，故太息以伸
出之。"指出心气可影响肺气，引起气道不利而胸闷、短气。

　　《诸病源候论•乏气候》说："夫虚极之人，营卫减耗，脏腑虚
弱，气行不足，所以呼吸短气。"心主营卫，营卫减耗，多含心气虚
衰。再及宗气，致使气弱，吐纳不及，故呼吸频率加快而气短。

《诸病源候论•少气候》说："此由脏气不足故也。肺主于气，而通呼吸，脏气不足，则呼吸微弱而少气。"这里的脏气泛指五脏之气，理应包含心气不足，影响于肺，而致呼吸短少。

Summary of Ancestral Qì Debility

1. Ancestral Qì Failing to Be in Charge of Breathing
 	
   Chest oppression and shortage of qì, short and discontinuous breathing or hasty rapid breathing, inability to lie down flat
2. External Discharge of Ancestral Qì
 	
   Apex of the heart beating so strongly that it is visible through the clothing

宗气衰少
不司呼吸 —— 胸闷少气、气短不续、或呼吸急促、不能平卧。 宗气外泄 —— 心尖搏动应衣。

Further Progressions

When the pathomechanism of heart qì vacuity advances one step further, it is involved in pathomechanisms such as heart yáng qì debility, dual vacuity of heart qì and blood, dual vacuity of heart qì and yīn or dual vacuity of heart qì and lung qì.

Heart Yáng Qì Debility

When heart qì vacuity is prolonged and the patient fails to recover, qì vacuity affects yáng. When yáng qì is damaged, it can develop into debility of the yáng qì of the heart. This condition is accompanied by heart palpitations and shortness of breath, and one may also observe cold signs such as chest pain, physical cold, and cool limbs.

Dual Vacuity of Heart Qì and Blood

Heart qì vacuity causes qì transformation failure and failure of qì to engender blood. This can result in heart blood vacuity, which may progress to dual vacuity of heart qì and blood. This manifests in heart palpitations and shortness of breath, as well as signs of dual vacuity of qì and blood, such as a pale face and pale lips and tongue.

Dual Vacuity of Heart Qì and Yīn

Heart qì vacuity causes qì to fail to form liquids; this results in an insufficiency of fluids. This, in turn, gives rise to heart yīn vacuity, creating dual vacuity of heart qì and yīn. Here, one can observe heart palpitations and shortness of breath, as well as pathoconditions of heart vexation, sleeplessness, and vexing heat in the five hearts.

Dual Vacuity of Heart Qì and Lung Qì

The heart governs the blood and vessels, and ancestral qì assists the heart in moving the blood. If there is prolonged insufficiency of heart qì, the ancestral qì also becomes vacuous, reducing the ability to breathe. This progression causes vacuity of lung qì, which forms the pathomechanism of heart and lung qì vacuity. Here, the patient will suffer from heart palpitations and fearful throbbing, in conjunction with chest oppression, shortness of breath, and cough and panting. Because the heart and lungs are linked together so closely, the vast majority of cases of heart qì vacuity also present with the pathomechanism of lung qì vacuity. Thus, these two pathomechanisms tend to present simultaneously.

心气虚的病机进一步发展，可形成心的阳气虚衰，心的气血两虚，心的气阴两虚，心肺气虚等病机。

心的阳气虚衰：心气虚日久不愈，气虚及阳,阳气受损，可发展成心的阳气虚衰。在心悸气短的同时，又见胸痛，形寒肢冷等寒象。

心的气血两虚：心气虚，气化无能，气不生血，可引起为心血虚，进而形成心的气血两虚。既见心悸气短，又见面唇舌淡等气血两虚之象。

心的气阴两虚：心气虚，气不化津，津液不足，可引起为心阴虚，进而形成心的气阴两虚。既见心悸气短，又见心烦失眠，五心烦热等症。

心肺气虚：心主血脉，宗气助心行血，心气不足，日久宗气亦虚，呼吸功能衰退，进而引起肺气虚弱，形成心肺气虚的病机。病人既有心悸怔忡，同时伴见胸闷气短咳喘等症。由于心肺关系十分密切，实际上大部分心气虚者，都可兼见肺气虚的病机，两种病机容易同时并存。

Chapter Nine

Heart Yáng Vacuity

The *Huáng Dì Nèi Jīng* ("The Yellow Emperor's Inner Canon") contains phrases such as "the heart and stomach engender cold" (*Sù Wèn*, "Plain Questions" # 74), "Great Treatise on the Essentials of Supreme Truth"), and "causing a person [to have] heart cold" (*Sù Wèn*, "Plain Questions"), "Treatise on Needling Heat [Conditions]"). However, these phrases do not yet formally name the pathomechanism of "heart yáng vacuity."

A later text, the *Qiān Jīn Yào Fāng* ("A Thousand Gold Pieces Prescriptions"), mentions the concept of "heart vacuity cold," based on a description from the *Mài Jīng* ("The Pulse Canon"). With the *Qiān Jīn Yào Fāng* ("A Thousand Gold Pieces Prescriptions") as their foundation, the texts *Shèng Jì Zǒng Lù* ("Sages' Salvation Records"), *Jì Shēng Fāng* ("Formulas for Saving Lives"), and *Dān Xī Shǒu Jìng* ("Dān-Xī's Hand Mirror") complement the discussion. The *Jì Shēng Fāng* ("Formulas for Saving Lives") contains the most comprehensive discussion, in the chapter "Discussing the Treatment of Heart and Small Intestine Vacuity and Repletion." It states:

> "Regarding their vacuity, when they are vacuous, cold is generated. Cold causes vacuity and scantiness of blood in the vessels, which manifests as occasional excessive fear, unhappiness, fulminant pain in the heart and abdomen, occasional spitting of clear drool, distention and fullness in the heart and diaphragm, forgetfulness and excessive fright, dreams of taking flight, a departing and scattered essence-spirit, and a floating and vacuous pulse. These are the symptoms of vacuity cold."

This quotation points out that heart vacuity cold can deprive the blood vessels of warmth and deprive the essence-spirit of nourishment.

The most clear early discussion of the pathomechanism of heart yáng vacuity is by Zhāng Jǐng-Yuè. In the *Jìng Yuè Quán Shū* ("Jǐng-Yuè's Complete Compendium"), "Records of Faithful Transmission," in the "Chapter on Vacuity and Repletion," he points out, "As for heart vacuity, it means yáng vacuity and excessive sorrow."

The commentary of the *Lèi Jīng* ("The Classified Canon") makes the following statement in reference to the *Sù Wèn* ("Plain Questions") chapter on "Methods of Treating Visceral Qì According to the Seasons": "The region between the chest, abdomen, lumbus, and rib-sides is reached by the hand lesser yīn and reverting yīn vessels. In cases of heart vacuity, yáng will be vacuous and counterflow qì will fail to move, thereby causing an enlarged chest and abdomen."

Both of the above statements pinpoint the pathomechanism of heart yáng vacuity. In the contemporary text *Pú Fǔ Zhōu Yī Liáo Jīng Yàn* ("Pú Fǔ-Zhōu's Medical Experience"), in the chapter on "Identifying Patterns and Seeking Roots," the pathomechanism of heart yáng vacuity is described succinctly from a clinical angle: "Heart yáng vacuity causes susceptibility to fear and unhappiness, spontaneous sweating, heart palpitations, apprehensive stirring, and lack of sleep." Ever since this text, the use of the pathomechanism of heart yáng vacuity has become widespread.

Heart yáng vacuity can result from many factors. It may arise from advanced heart qì vacuity. It can also be caused by enduring insufficiency of heart yīn if the yīn damage affects yáng. Other factors that lead to debility of heart yáng include severe damage to yáng by fulminant disease and congenital constitutional insufficiency. Inappropriate convalescence and lack of treatment or inappropriate treatment may also result in devitalized heart yáng. Finally, heart yáng vacuity may arise from the passage of disorders from other bowels and viscera.

Essentially, the pathomechanism of heart yáng vacuity revolves around insufficiency of yáng qì and the internal generation of vacuity cold. Yáng qì is responsible for such important physiological functions as warming and nourishing the essence-spirit, promoting the free flow of blood in the vessels, and quickening and transforming fluids. When heart yáng is debilitated, it fails to perform its functions of warming, propelling, steaming, soaring, and transforming qì. This pathomechanism can manifest as a heart spirit deprived of nourishment (including fulminant desertion of heart yáng), heart vessels deprived of warmth, insecurity of heart yáng, and water collection and liquid obstruction.

心阳虚

　　《黄帝内经》有"心胃生寒"（《素问•至真要大论》），"令人心寒"（《素问•刺热论》）等提法，未正式提出"心阳虚"病机的名称。其后《千金要方》根据《脉经》的论述，提出了"心虚寒"的概念。《圣济总录》、《济生方》、《丹溪手镜》在《千金要方》的基础上作了补充，特别是《济生方•心小肠虚实论治》论述最全面，是书说："方其虚，虚则生寒，寒则血脉虚少，时多恐畏，情绪不乐，心腹暴痛，时唾清涎，心膈胀满，好忘多惊，梦寐飞扬，精神离散，其脉浮而虚，是虚寒之候也。"指出心虚寒可引起血脉失温和精神失养。最为明确提出心阳虚的病机首推张景岳，他在《景岳全书•传忠录•虚实篇》指出："心虚者，阳虚而多悲"。又在《类经》注释并引申《素问•藏气法时论》时说："胸腹腰胁之间皆手少阴、厥阴之脉所及，心虚则阳虚，而逆气不行，故为胸腹大。"两处皆直接点明心阳虚的病机。近代《蒲辅周医疗经验•辨证求本》一书中从临床的角度对心阳虚病机作了准确描述，认为"心阳虚，则善恐不乐，自汗，心悸，惕惕然而动，少寐。"至此之后，心阳虚的病机已被普遍运用。

心阳虚可由心气虚进一步发展而成；或由心阴不足，久而不愈，阴损及阳而致；或由暴病伤阳，心阳严重损耗；或因先天禀赋不足，引起心阳虚衰；或因病后调养失宜，或失治误治，导致心阳不振；或由其它脏腑病证的传变，波及心阳。

心阳虚的病机本质在于阳气不足，虚寒内生。阳气有温养精神，流通血脉，活化津液等重要生理功能。故当心阳虚衰，温煦、推动、蒸腾、气化等功能失职时，其病机可表现为心神失养（包括心阳暴脱），心脉失温、心阳不固和水停津阻等几个方面。

9.1 Heart Spirit Deprived of Nourishment

The *Sù Wèn* ("Plain Questions"), "Treatise on Vital Qì Connecting to Heaven" states, "The essence of yang qì nourishes the spirit." This quotation explains that yáng qì is the material foundation for mental activity. The heart governs the spirit-mind, and the degree of exuberance, debility, strength, or weakness of heart yáng is linked closely to the activity of the spirit-mind.

Various factors can damage heart yáng and cause the heart spirit to be deprived of nourishment. Depending on the severity of the vacuity detriment, different states of the spirit-mind will manifest. Commonly seen pathological changes include a devitalized essence-spirit, a disquieted heart spirit, or in extreme cases, fulminant desertion of heart yáng.

心神失养

"阳气者，精则养神"（《素问•生气通天论》），说明阳气是精神活动的物质基础。心主神志，心阳的盛衰强弱，与人的神志活动有密切关系。各种原因致使心阳受伤，均会引起心神失养，并随其虚损程度的差异表现不同的神志状态。常见的病机变化是精神不振、心神不安，甚至引起心阳暴脱。

9.1.1 Devitalized Essence-Spirit

In its normal state, heart yáng is full and able to warm and promote free flow of the blood to provide nourishment to the heart spirit. Thus, the essence-spirit is vitalized and the heart is able to "control substances." In heart yáng insufficiency, qì and blood fail to supply nourishment and vitality to the heart spirit. This will manifest in mental listlessness, lassitude of the spirit with desire for sleep, an indifferent expression, emotional depression, or somnolence with no strength to speak.

The *Shāng Hán Lùn* ("On Cold Damage"), in "Lesser Yīn Channel Pattern Identification and Treatment," states, "In lesser yīn disorders, the pulse will be faint and thin with a desire only to sleep." Lesser yīn disorders belong to the pattern of heart and kidney yáng vacuity. A "desire only to sleep" refers to a condition of heart yáng insufficiency with vacuity of the heart spirit. It manifests with listlessness of essence-spirit, utter exhaustion, lack of strength to speak or move, and a state resembling neither sleep nor wakefulness. This condition should be treated by supplementing heart yáng and vitalizing the essence-spirit. An appropriate formula is Ginseng and Aconite Decoction (*shēn fù tāng*) from the *Fù Rén Liáng Fāng* ("Good Remedies for Women"), with the addition of astragalus.

Ginseng and Aconite Decoction (参附汤 *shēn fù tāng*)
rén shēn (人参 Ginseng Radix, ginseng)
fù zǐ (附子 Aconiti Radix Lateralis Praeparata, aconite)
Plus:
huáng qí (黄芪 Astragali Radix, astragalus)

精神不振

正常生理状况下，心阳充沛，能温通血液，奉养心神，则精神振奋，心能"任物"。若心阳不足，气血失供，心神失养，不能振奋，则表现为精神较差、或萎靡不振、神倦欲寐、表情淡漠、情绪不乐、嗜卧懒言等症。如《伤寒论•辨少阴脉证并治》云："少阴之为病，脉微细，但欲寐也。"少阴病为心肾阳虚证，"但欲寐"即是心阳不足，心神虚弱，而表现的精神萎靡、疲惫不堪、懒言懒动、似睡非睡的状态。治宜补养心阳，振奋精神。方用《妇人良方》参附汤（人参、附子）加黄芪。

9.1.2 Disquieted Heart Spirit

In most patients suffering from heart yáng vacuity, the loss of nourishment to the essence-spirit manifests as insufficient spirit-qì and essence-spirit debility. Heart yáng vacuity may also cause an inability to warm and move qì and blood to nourish the essence-spirit. This causes the spirit to fail to keep to its abode. Thus, at the time when one should fall asleep, the spirit and ethereal souls wander externally. This results in fidgetiness whether lying or up, insomnia, and excessive dreaming. Moreover, since the heart spirit is deprived of nourishment, memory is poor. This produces forgetfulness and negligence, heart vacuity and lack of courage, and susceptibility to fright when encountering things. It should be treated by supplementing heart yáng and quieting the heart spirit. For a formula, use Cinnamon Twig, Licorice, Dragon Bone, and Oyster Shell Decoction (*guì zhī gān cǎo lóng gǔ mǔ lì tāng*) from the *Shāng Hán Lùn* ("On Cold Damage").

Cinnamon Twig, Licorice, Dragon Bone, and Oyster Shell Decoction
(桂枝甘草龙骨牡蛎汤 *guì zhī gān cǎo lóng gǔ mǔ lì tāng*)

guì zhī (桂枝 Cinnamomi Ramulus, cinnamon twig)
gān cǎo (甘草 Glycyrrhizae Radix, licorice)
lóng gǔ (龙骨 Mastodi Ossis Fossilia, dragon bone)
mǔ lì (牡蛎 Ostreae Concha, oyster shell)

心神不安

大部分心阳虚的患者，精神失养，表现为神气不足，精神衰败。亦有心阳虚，不能温运气血，濡养精神，使心神不能内守，应当安眠入睡时，却神魂外游，而致卧起不安、失眠多梦。并因心神失养，不能记忆，而好忘遗事，心虚胆小而遇事易惊。治宜补心阳，安心神。方用《伤寒论》桂枝甘草龙骨牡蛎汤（桂枝、甘草、龙骨、牡蛎）。

Literature Review of Disquieted Heart Spirit

📖 *Jì Shēng Fāng* ("Formulas for Saving Lives"), "On the Treatment of Heart and Small Intestine Vacuity and Repletion"

"As for vacuity, vacuity engenders cold; cold causes vacuity of the blood in the vessels, occasional profuse fear, and unhappiness… forgetfulness and profuse dreaming, and dreams of flying."

In heart yáng vacuity cold, heart yáng is insufficient; yáng is vacuous and blood is scant. The heart spirit is deprived of nourishment, the essence-spirit is devitalized, and there is forgetfulness and unquiet sleep.

文献评述

《济生方•心与小肠虚实论治》说："方其虚，虚则生寒，寒则血脉虚少，时多恐畏，情绪不乐，…好忘多梦，梦寐飞扬。"心的虚寒，心阳不足，阳虚血少，心神失养，精神不振，健忘遗事，睡眠不安。

9.1.3　Fulminant Desertion of Heart Yáng

When heart yáng has sustained severe and critical damage to the point of extreme debility, it can result in fulminant desertion and collapse of yáng qì. This may be caused by a sudden disease that damages yáng or by the progression of yáng vacuity over a prolonged period of time. If the heart spirit is severely wounded, it becomes disquieted and insecure. Instead of keeping to its abode, it will stray outward, giving rise to the pathomechanism of fulminant desertion of heart yáng.

In the initial stages, one can observe the symptoms of heart vexation and agitation. This occurs because fulminant desertion of heart yáng causes the heart spirit to be deprived of nourishment, which leads to vexation, derangement, and lack of tranquility. It should be treated by supplementing heart yáng and eliminating vexation and agitation. For a formula, use Counterflow Cold Decoction (*sì nì tāng*) from the *Shāng Hán Lùn* ("On Cold Damage").

Counterflow Cold Decoction (四逆汤 *sì nì tāng*)

fù zǐ (附子 Aconiti Radix Lateralis Praeparata, aconite)
gān jiāng (干姜 Zingiberis Rhizoma, dried ginger)
zhì gān cǎo (炙甘草 Glycyrrhizae Radix cum Liquido Fricta, mix-fried licorice)

The *Shāng Hán Lùn* ("On Cold Damage"), in "Reverting Yīn Vessel Pattern Identification and Treatment," states, "In cold damage disorders, the pulse is faint and reverting. If, by the seventh or eighth day, the skin is cold and the person is agitated without a single moment of peace, this is visceral reversal." In this instance, the faint pulse indicates heart yáng vacuity causing forceless movement. The agitation and harassment are due to heart yáng debility causing the heart spirit to be deprived of nourishment. Thus, the spirit is disquiet and frequently stirs.

If this condition is followed by the departure and scattering of the essence-spirit and the outward desertion of spirit-qì, one will observe severe symptoms of fulminant desertion of heart yáng. The symptoms include abstraction of the spirit-mind, unclear consciousness, coma, or loss of consciousness. At this time, one should drastically supplement heart yáng to return yáng and stem counterflow. For a formula, use Ginseng, Aconite, Dragon Bone, and Oyster Shell (*shēn fù lóng lǐ tāng*) from the *Shì Yī Dé Xiào Fāng* ("Effective Formulas From a Family Tradition") to return yáng and stem desertion. If the condition advances further, the heartbeat will stop, the pulse will expire, qì will desert, and death will follow.

Ginseng, Aconite, Dragon Bone, and Oyster Shell (参附龙牡汤 *shēn fù lóng lǐ tāng*)

rén shēn (人参 Ginseng Radix, ginseng)
fù zǐ (附子 Aconiti Radix Lateralis Praeparata, aconite)
lóng gǔ (龙骨 Mastodi Ossis Fossilia, dragon bone)
mǔ lì (牡蛎 Ostreae Concha, oyster shell)

心阳暴脱

暴病伤阳，或心阳虚进一步发展，迁延日久，心阳受到严重损伤而致衰极，阳气暴脱而亡失，心神重创，不能安泰固守于内而外越，则引起心阳暴脱的病机。初起可见心烦躁扰不宁之症。是因心阳暴脱，心神失养，烦乱蠢动，不得宁静所致。治宜补心阳，除烦躁。方用《伤寒论》四逆汤（附子、干姜、炙甘草）。如《伤寒论·辨厥阴病脉证并治》："伤寒，脉微而厥，至七八日，肤冷，其人躁无暂安时者，此为藏厥。"其中脉微乃心阳虚，无力鼓动。躁扰不宁，是心阳虚衰，心神失养，神不安泰，时时欲动，心绪难宁。随即引起精神离散，神气外脱，而见神志恍惚，意识不清，昏迷不省人事等心阳暴脱的危重症状。此时当务之急是大补心阳，回阳救逆，用《世医得效方》参附龙牡汤（人参、附子、龙骨、牡蛎）回阳固脱，可挽救其万一。否则病情进一步发展，引起心跳骤停，脉绝气脱，而致死亡。

Literature Review of Fulminant Desertion of Heart Yáng

📖 *Qiān Jīn Yào Fāng* ("A Thousand Gold Pieces Prescriptions"), "Heart Vacuity Cold"

"When the heart feels cold in conjunction with abstraction, it is heart vacuity cold."

This quotation explains that in cases of heart yáng vacuity, the essence-spirit is deprived of nourishment and the heart loses its ability to govern the essence-spirit, thoughts, and consciousness. This results in abstraction and an unclear spirit-mind.

📖 *Tĭ Rén Huì Biān* ("A Corpus on the Body"), "The Nature of Medicinals in the Heart Viscus"

"Cases of vacuity cold present with timidity, fear, susceptibility to fright, forgetfulness, and abstraction."

This quotation points out that heart yáng debility causes the heart spirit to be deprived of nourishment. Thus, it fails to govern thought and consciousness, which can result in forgetfulness and abstraction of the essence-spirit.

📖 *Líng Shū* ("The Magic Pivot"), "Visiting of Evil"

"The heart is the great governor of the five viscera and six bowels and the abode of the essence-spirit. When the heart is damaged, the spirit leaves. When the spirit leaves, death follows."

Heart yáng is the primary force for stimulating mental activity in the human body. When heart yáng is in a state of extreme debility, yáng fails to be constrained by yīn; the heart spirit flies astray, the essence-spirit departs and scatters, and the vitality of the five organs expires. This results in clouding of the spirit or death. At the same time, one may see manifestations of yáng collapse, such as dripping great sweat, counterflow cold in the four limbs, and a pale white facial complexion.

文献评述

《千金要方•心虚寒》云："心如寒，恍惚，曰心虚寒也。"说明心阳虚，精神失养，心失去主管精神、思维、意识的功能，故致神志恍惚不清。

《体仁汇编•心藏药性》说："虚寒者怯怕多惊，健忘恍惚。"也指出心阳虚衰，心神失养，不主思维、意识，可致健忘遗事，精神恍惚。

《灵枢•邪客篇》说："心者五脏六腑之大主也，精神之所舍也。…心伤则神去，神去则死矣。"心阳是激发人体精神活动的主要动力，心阳衰极，阳失阴恋，心神飞越，精神离散，五脏生机已绝，故神昏而死。同时可见大汗淋漓，四肢逆冷，面色苍白等亡阳表现。

Summary of Heart Spirit Deprived of Nourishment

1. **Devitalized Essence-Spirit**

   Poor essence-spirit, possibly with listlessness and lassitude of the spirit and desire to sleep, indifferent expression, unhappiness, or somnolence with no strength to speak

2. **Disquieted Heart Spirit**

   Fidgetiness whether lying or up, sleeplessness and profuse dreaming, or forgetfulness and susceptibility to fright when encountering things

3. **Fulminant Desertion of Heart Yáng**

   Heart spirit deprived of nourishment: Heart vexation, agitation, and derangement

   Scattering and desertion of spirit-qì: Abstraction of the spirit-mind, unclear consciousness, coma or loss of consciousness

   Heart spirit flying astray: Racing or stopping of the heartbeat, pulse expiry and qì desertion leading to death

心神失养

精神不振 —— 精神较差、或萎靡不振、神倦欲眠。表情淡漠、情绪不乐、嗜卧懒言。

心神不安 —— 卧起不安、失眠多梦。好忘遗事、遇事易惊。

心阳暴脱

  心神失养 —— 心烦躁乱。

  神气散脱 —— 神志恍惚，意识不清，昏迷不省。

  心神飞越 —— 心跳骤停，脉绝气脱，引起死亡。

9.2 Heart Vessels Deprived of Warmth

The *Sù Wèn* ("Plain Questions") text, in the "Treatise on the Engenderment of the Five Viscera," states, "The heart is connected to the vessels" and "all blood belongs to the heart." These statements clarify the close relationship of the heart with the blood and the vessels. In this context, heart yáng has a warming and propelling function; it is of great significance in maintaining the normal activity of the blood and vessels. When heart yáng is debilitated, its ability to warm and move the blood in the vessels is reduced. This pathomechanism manifests in vessels losing warmth and nourishment and in congealing cold with blood stasis.

心脉失温

《素问·五藏生成篇》曰："心之合脉也"，"诸血者皆属于心"，说明心与血和脉有密切的关系。其中心阳对血和脉有温煦、推动作用，对维持血脉正常生理活动有重要的意义。心阳虚衰，减少对血脉的温运，则会出现脉失温养和寒凝血瘀的病机变化。

9.2.1 Vessels Deprived of Warmth and Nourishment

The *Sù Wèn* ("Plain Questions"), in the "Treatise on the Six Periods and Visceral Manifestation," states, "The heart is the root of life. … Its bloom is in the face and its fullness is in the blood vessels." In its normal physiological condition, heart yáng warms and propels forcefully, causing blood and qì to be effulgent and the blood vessels to flow smoothly.

When the blood in the face is full, the face, lips, and tongue are red and moist and full of vitality and sheen. When blood nourishes the body of the heart, the movement of the heart is regular and the pulse is calm and leisurely, harmonious, moderate, and forceful. When blood and construction reach the four limbs, the hands and feet are warm and move freely. When blood is distributed throughout the body, the body is comfortably warm all over and essence-spirit is abundant.

If heart yáng is debilitated, blood and qì fail to nourish the body of the heart; thus, the heart viscus contracts and lacks strength. It is unable to move blood throughout the body and only accelerates its beat within the heart viscus itself. Because it lacks strength for warming and propelling, the heart blood is simultaneously reduced, the heart spirit is deprived of nourishment, and the heart spirit becomes disquiet. This can result in pathoconditions with flusteredness, fatigue of the heart, emptiness in the heart, or palpitations below the heart. It should be treated by supplementing yáng qì while nourishing the heart and quieting the spirit. For a formula, use Ginseng and Aconite Decoction (*shēn fù tāng*) from the *Fù Rén Liáng Fāng* ("Good Remedies for Women"), with the addition of astragalus, cinnamon twig, polygala, root poria, and licorice.

Ginseng and Aconite Decoction (参附汤 *shēn fù tāng*)
rén shēn (人参 Ginseng Radix, ginseng)
fù zǐ (附子 Aconiti Radix Lateralis Praeparata, aconite)
Plus:
huáng qí (黄芪 Astragali Radix, astragalus)
guì zhī (桂枝 Cinnamomi Ramulus, cinnamon twig)
yuǎn zhì (远志 Polygalae Radix, polygala)
fú shén (茯神 Poria cum Pini Radice, root poria)
gān cǎo (甘草 Glycyrrhizae Radix, licorice)

If heart yáng is debilitated, it lacks strength for warming and moving. Qì and blood are thus unable to ascend to provide luxuriance to the face, and the blood vessels in the face, lips, and tongue are empty. When qì loses warmth and blood loses fullness, pathoconditions with a pale white or somber white facial complexion, pale-colored lips and tongue, or a lusterless facial complexion result. When yáng qì is unable to warm and nourish the head and eyes, the head will be clouded and the vision will be flowery. This should be treated by warming and nourishing heart yáng while supplementing qì and upraising. For a formula, use Astragalus and Aconite Decoction (*qí fù tāng*) from the *Chóng Dìng Yán Shì Jì Shēng Fāng* ("Revised Yan's Remedies for Curing All People"), in combination with Center-Supplementing Qì-Boosting Decoction (*bǔ zhōng yì qì tāng*) from the *Pí Wèi Lùn* ("On the Spleen and Stomach").

Astragalus and Aconite Decoction (芪附汤 *qí fù tāng*)

huáng qí (黄芪 Astragali Radix, astragalus)
fù zǐ (附子 Aconiti Radix Lateralis Praeparata, aconite)

Center-Supplementing Qì-Boosting Decoction (补中益气汤 *bǔ zhōng yì qì tāng*)

huáng qí (黄芪 Astragali Radix, astragalus)
rén shēn (人参 Ginseng Radix, ginseng)
dāng guī (当归 Angelicae Sinensis Radix, Chinese angelica)
chái hú (柴胡 Bupleuri Radix, bupleurum)
shēng má (升麻 Cimicifugae Rhizoma, cimicifuga)
bái zhú (白朮 Atractylodis Macrocephalae Rhizoma, white atractylodes)
gān cǎo (甘草 Glycyrrhizae Radix, licorice)

Irregularity of the heartbeat may result from the body of the heart being deprived of the warmth and nourishment of yáng qì; this manifests as a pulse that is skipping, bound, intermittent, or scattered. If heart yáng lacks strength, the vessel qì is unable to propel and uplift, causing the pulse to be slow and possibly either fine, faint, and forceless or fine, rapid, and forceless. This condition should be treated by warming and nourishing heart yáng while boosting qì to free the vessels. For a formula, use Ginseng and Aconite Decoction (*shēn fù tāng*) from the *Fù Rén Liáng Fāng* ("Good Remedies for Women"), with the addition of Chinese angelica, raw rehmannia, white peony, cinnamon twig, and mix-fried licorice.

Ginseng and Aconite Decoction (参附汤 *shēn fù tāng*)

rén shēn (人参 Ginseng Radix, ginseng)

fù zǐ (附子 Aconiti Radix Lateralis Praeparata, aconite)

Plus:

dāng guī (当归 Angelicae Sinensis Radix, Chinese angelica)

shēng dì huáng (生地黄 Rehmanniae Radix Exsiccata seu Recens, dried/fresh rehmannia)

bái sháo (白芍 Paeoniae Radix Alba, white peony)

guì zhī (桂枝 Cinnamomi Ramulus, cinnamon twig)

zhì gān cǎo (炙甘草 Glycyrrhizae Radix cum Liquido Fricta, mix-fried licorice)

The four limbs are the root of all yáng. If heart yáng is debilitated, cold is engendered from the inside and yáng qì is unable to follow the blood to warm the four limbs. If this occurs, the hands and feet will lack warmth, or there may be reversal cold of the four limbs. When the four limbs are deprived of nourishment, their function and activities are limited. This manifests in limp aching hands and feet that lack strength and move without spirit. The failure of heart yáng to warm qì and blood to reach the four limbs causes sensory disturbances, manifesting as numbness in the limbs. This should be treated by warming and freeing heart yáng while supplementing yáng qì. For a formula, use Chinese Angelica Counterflow Cold Decoction (*dāng guī sì nì tāng*) from the *Shāng Hán Lùn* ("On Cold Damage"), with the addition of astragalus and ginseng.

Chinese Angelica Counterflow Cold Decoction (当归四逆汤 *dāng guī sì nì tāng*)

guì zhī (桂枝 Cinnamomi Ramulus, cinnamon twig)

dāng guī (当归 Angelicae Sinensis Radix, Chinese angelica)

bái sháo (白芍 Paeoniae Radix Alba, white peony)

xīn yí (辛夷 Magnoliae Flos, magnolia flower)

mù tōng (木通 Akebiae Trifoliatae Caulis, trifoliate akebia)

dà zǎo (大枣 Jujubae Fructus, jujube)

zhì gān cǎo (炙甘草 Glycyrrhizae Radix cum Liquido Fricta, mix-fried licorice)

Plus:

huáng qí (黄芪 Astragali Radix, astragalus)

rén shēn (人参 Ginseng Radix, ginseng)

脉失温养

《素问•六节藏象论》说："心者，生之本也。…其华在面，其充在血脉。"正常生理状况下，心阳温煦，推动有力，则血气旺盛，血脉流畅。血液充盈于面，则颜面、唇舌红润，有生气、有光泽。血养心体，则心动有节，脉来从容，和缓有力；血营四肢，则手足温暖，运动自如。血布全身，则周身暖和，精神充沛。若心阳虚衰，血气不养于心体，心脏收缩乏力，不能鼓动血液运行全身，只得加快心脏搏动；同时又因温运乏力，心血减少，心神失养，心神不安，故可引起心慌、心累，心中空虚，心下悸动等症。治宜补养阳气，养心安神。方用《妇人良方》参附汤加黄芪、桂枝、远志、茯神、甘草。

若心阳虚衰，温运乏力，气血不能上荣于面，面部、唇舌血脉空虚，气失温煦、血失充盈，则为面色淡白或苍白，唇舌色淡，面色无华等症。阳气不能温养于头目，则头昏眼花。治宜温养心阳，补气升提。方用《重订严氏济生方》芪附汤（黄芪、附子）合《脾胃论》补中益气汤（黄芪、人参、当归、柴胡、升麻、白术、甘草）。或因心体失去阳气温养，搏动节律失调，脉象出现促、结、代、散等变化；或因心阳鼓动无力，脉气无以推动、升举，脉来迟慢，或细微无力，或细数无力。治宜温养心阳，益气通脉。方用《妇人良方》参附汤加当归、生地、白芍、桂枝、炙甘草。

四肢为诸阳之本，若心阳虚衰，寒从内生，阳气不能随血温煦四肢，则为手足不温或四肢厥冷；四肢失养，功能活动受限，则为手足酸软无力，运动失灵；不能温煦气血到达四肢，感觉障碍，则为肢体麻木不仁。治宜温通心阳，补益阳气。方用《伤寒论》当归四逆汤（桂枝、当归、白芍、细辛、木通、大枣、炙甘草）加黄芪、人参。

Literature Review of Vessels Deprived of Warmth and Nourishment

📖 *Shāng Hán Míng Lǐ Lùn* ("The Clear Rationale of Cold Damage"), "Palpitations"

> "In cases of qì vacuity, there is internal weakness of yáng qì, emptiness below the heart, and palpitations from the internal stirring of right qì."

Palpitations below the heart are a pathology ascribed to the heart. An internal debility of yáng qì throughout the body is bound to influence the heart. When heart yáng is weak and loses its ability to warm and nourish, abnormal stirring of the heart will result. Therefore, the pathoconditions of heart palpitations and emptiness below the heart arise.

📖 *Yī Zōng Jīn Jiàn* ("The Golden Mirror of Orthodox Medicine"), "Revised Commentary on the *Shāng Hán Lùn* ("On Cold Damage")"

> "In cases where sweating is followed by fright palpitations below the heart, it means that the yáng inside the heart is vacuous."

Yang qì forces the fluids to the outside, causing sweating. When sweating is excessive, the yáng qì in the heart will invariably sustain damage; heart yáng will be vacuous and the heart spirit will be deprived of nourishment. This gives rise to heart palpitations.

📖 *Bǐ Huā Yī Jìng* ("*Bǐ Huā* Medical Mirror"), "Heart Section"

> "Cold in the heart invariably manifests as a slow inch pulse on the left side."

Cold in the heart means heart yáng vacuity. The left inch pulse is ascribed to the heart; here the heart pulse is slow. This quotation explains that heart yáng vacuity can cause a slow heart pulse.

📖 *Tǐ Rén Huì Biān* ("A Corpus on the Body"), "The Nature of Medicinals in the Heart Viscus"

> "In cases of vacuity cold, there will be timidity and profuse palpitations…the pulse will invariably be soggy, fine, slow, and vacuous."

Vacuity cold in the entire body includes heart yáng debility. When heart yáng is vacuous, the heart spirit is deprived of nourishment; this can result in heart palpitations. Because there is a loss of warmth and movement, the movement in the pulse is without strength; this manifests as a pulse that is soggy, fine, slow, and vacuous.

📖 *Shèng Jì Zǒng Lù* ("Sages' Salvation Records"), "Cold Damage Reversal"

> "When a cold damage patient suffers from counterflow cold in the hands and feet, it is called reversal. This is caused by debility of yáng qì and exuberance of yīn qì. When yīn qì is exuberant, the yáng vessels counterflow and fail to flow into the four limbs. This causes counterflow cold."

📖 *Jǐng Yuè Quán Shū* ("Jǐng-Yuè's Complete Compendium"), "Schema of Miscellaneous Patterns," "Reversal Counterflow"

> "All cases of cold reversal invariably present with clear coolness in the four limbs and a pulse that is deep, faint, and not rapid, or else rapid but lacking in strength."

The two passages above do not yet clearly indicate the situation of heart yáng debility. However, by stating that "when yīn qì is exuberant, the yáng vessels counterflow and fail to flow into the four limbs," with a pulse manifesting as "deep, faint, and not rapid, or else rapid but lacking in strength," they obviously relate the state of extreme heart yáng vacuity to exuberant cold that is causing contraction in the channels and vessels. The cold causes retraction, blockage, and inhibition in the blood vessels.

Another possibility is that the propelling action of heart yáng lacks strength, causing yáng qì and blood to fail to reach the four limbs. In this case, one can observe the manifestation of the limbs being cold as ice. When heart yáng is vacuous, it is unable to propel the blood and warm and nourish the entire body. This can result in a generalized aversion to cold and liking for warmth, lying down in a curled-up posture, and a fatigued spirit.

文献评述

《伤寒明理论·悸》说："其气虚者，由阳气内弱，心下空虚，正气内动而为悸也。"心下悸动，是属心的病变，全身阳气内衰，一定影响于心，心阳虚弱，失于温养，才能引起心动异常，而致心悸、心下空虚等症发生。

《医宗金鉴·订正伤寒论注》更明确指出："发汗后心下惊悸者，乃虚其心中之阳"。阳气逼迫津液外出而为汗，发汗过度，心中阳气必然受到损伤，心阳虚，心神失养，从而引起心悸。

《笔花医镜·心部》说："心之寒，脉左寸必迟。"心之寒，即是心阳虚。左寸脉属心，系指心脉迟慢。说明心阳虚，可致心脉迟慢。

《体仁汇编·心脏药性》说："虚寒者，怯怕多悸，…脉必濡细迟虚。"全身虚寒，包括心阳虚衰。心阳虚，心神失养，可致心悸；失于温运、推动，运脉无力，可致濡细迟虚。

《圣济总录·伤寒厥》云："伤寒病手足逆冷，其名曰厥。此因阳气衰阴气盛，阴盛则阳脉逆而不通于四肢，所以逆冷。"

《景岳全书·杂证谟·厥逆》亦说："凡寒厥，必四肢清凉，脉沉微不数，或虽数而无力。"这里虽未明确指出为心阳虚衰，但"阴盛则阳脉逆而不通于四肢"，脉见"沉微不数，或虽数无力"，显然均系心阳虚极，寒盛经脉收引，血脉缩闭而不利；或心阳推动无力，阳气、血液不达于四肢，才能见到肢冷如冰的表现。心阳虚，不能推动血液，温养全身，可致全身畏寒喜暖，蜷卧神疲。

Summary of Vessels Deprived of Warmth and Nourishment

1. Failure to Warm the Heart

    Flusteredness, a fatigued heart, stirring palpitations below the heart, a pulse that is fine, rapid, and forceless
2. Failure to Warm the Head and Face

    Clouded head and flowery vision, pale white and lusterless facial complexion, pale-colored lips and tongue
3. Failure to Warm the Vessels

    A pulse that is skipping, bound, intermittent, or scattered, possibly slow, or possibly fine, faint, and without strength
4. Failure to Warm the Four Limbs

    Reversal cold in the four limbs, limp aching hands and feet, spiritless movement, numbness in the limbs

脉失温养

不温于心 —— 心慌、心累，心下悸动，脉细数乏力。

不温于头面—— 头昏眼花，面色淡白无华，唇舌色淡。

不温于脉 —— 促、结、代、散或迟慢，或细微无力。

不温四肢 —— 四肢厥冷，手足酸软，运动失灵，肢体麻木。

9.2.2   Congealing Cold with Blood Stasis

气为阳，血为阴，阳主动，阴主静，阳气推动而血行，阳气衰而血
泣。正如《素问•调经论》所云："血气者，喜温而恶寒，寒则泣而
不能流，温则消而去之。"心主血脉，血能正常营运，全赖心阳推
动，才能循环无端，周流不息。心阳虚衰，寒从中生，寒主凝滞可
使血泣，阳失推动可使血运迟慢，均可导致寒凝血瘀之病机。

Qì is yáng and blood is yīn. Yáng governs movement, yīn governs stillness. When yáng qì propels, the blood moves. If yáng qì is debilitated, the blood chokes and gets stuck. The *Sù Wèn* ("Plain Questions") chapter, "On Regulating the Channels" states, "Blood and qì like warmth and are averse to cold. When cold is present, they choke and cannot flow. Warmth disperses and eliminates."

The heart governs the blood and vessels. The normal ability of the blood to move construction depends entirely on the propelling activity of heart yáng to circulate endlessly. When heart yáng is debilitated, cold arises from the center. Cold governs congealing; thus, it can cause the blood to choke and become stuck and become stuck. When yáng fails to propel, the movement of blood slows. All these circumstances can lead to the pathomechanism of congealing cold with blood stasis.

The *Yī Lǐ Zhēn Chuán* ("True Transmission of Medical Principles"), in the chapter, "Inquiry on Yáng Vacuity Pathoconditions," states, "The heart is the commander of qì. When heart yáng is supplemented, lung qì becomes effulgent." This statement shows how closely related the exuberance or debility of lung qì is to the state of heart yáng.

When heart yáng is debilitated, lung qì is damaged, yáng qì in the chest is devitalized, and qì and blood congeal in the chest. This congests chest qì and leads to chest impediment. Commonly observed manifestations include chest fullness, hasty panting, shortness and inhibition of breath, tautness and pain in the chest and back, bound qì, and coughing and spitting.

The main emphasis in this pathomechanism should be on the debility of yáng qì in the heart and lungs, rather than the congestion from phlegm turbidity. In treatment, one should employ supplementing methods. Appropriate treatment should warm and free heart yáng while dissipating binds and opening impediment. For a formula, choose Ginseng Decoction (*rén shēn tāng*) from the *Jīn Guì Yào Lüè* ("Essential Prescriptions of the Golden Coffer"), with the addition of cinnamon twig, apricot kernel, platycodon, unripe bitter orange, and tangerine peel. This will warm the spleen and heart, supplement heart yáng, and dissipate binds to open the impediment.

Ginseng Decoction (人参汤 *rén shēn tāng*)
rén shēn (人参 Ginseng Radix, ginseng)
gān jiāng (干姜 Zingiberis Rhizoma, dried ginger)
bái zhú (白朮 Atractylodis Macrocephalae Rhizoma, white atractylodes)
gān cǎo (甘草 Glycyrrhizae Radix, licorice)
Plus:
guì zhī (桂枝 Cinnamomi Ramulus, cinnamon twig)
xìng rén (杏仁 Armeniacae Semen, apricot kernel)
jié gěng (桔梗 Platycodonis Radix, platycodon)
zhǐ shí (枳实 Aurantii Fructus Immaturus, unripe bitter orange)
chén pí (陈皮 Citri Reticulatae Pericarpium, tangerine peel)

If heart yáng is debilitated and cold congeals the blood vessels in the body of the heart, the movement of blood will be slow, rough, and congested; this will result in heart pain. If the congealing cold and blood stasis is mild, it will cause stabbing pain in the heart [region] and chest that stretches to the back; this will recur repeatedly and there will be a liking for warmth and an aversion to coolness. It should be treated by warming yáng and boosting qì while quickening blood and transforming stasis. For a formula, use Ginseng and Aconite Decoction (*shēn fù tāng*) from the *Fù Rén Liáng Fāng* ("Good Remedies for Women"), with the addition of cinnamon twig, Chinese angelica, chuanxiong, salvia, curcuma, and licorice.

Ginseng and Aconite Decoction (参附汤 *shēn fù tāng*)
rén shēn (人参 Ginseng Radix, ginseng)
fù zǐ (附子 Aconiti Radix Lateralis Praeparata, aconite)
Plus:
guì zhī (桂枝 Cinnamomi Ramulus, cinnamon twig)
dāng guī (当归 Angelicae Sinensis Radix, Chinese angelica)
chuān xiōng (川芎 Chuanxiong Rhizoma, chuanxiong)
dān shēn (丹参 Salviae Miltiorrhizae Radix, salvia)
yù jīn (郁金 Curcumae Radix, curcuma)
gān cǎo (甘草 Glycyrrhizae Radix, licorice)

In more serious cases of congealing cold and blood stasis, the obstruction of the heart vessels will be severe. Here, the patient will suffer from sudden attacks of severe pain in the heart; the pain is aggravated by exposure to cold and is relieved by warmth. There will be heart pain stretching through to the back or back pain stretching through to the heart, along with counterflow cold of the extremities. The face and lips will be blue-green, purple, or dark, and the nails will be dark purple. The tongue body will be dark with stasis macules and stasis speckles on the tip and sides, with exposed sublingual network vessels. The pulse will be either skipping, bound, or intermittent, or else faint and fine on the verge of expiry. This should be treated by warming yáng and quickening blood while expelling cold and relieving pain. For a formula, use Aconite Main Tuber and Halloysite Pill (*wū tóu chì shí zhī wán*) from the *Jīn Guì Yào Lüè* ("Essential Prescriptions of the Golden Coffer"), with the addition of ginseng, cinnamon twig, Chinese angelica, red peony, and mix-fried licorice.

Aconite Main Tuber and Halloysite Pill (乌头赤石脂丸 *wū tóu chì shí zhī wán*)
wū tóu (乌头 Aconiti Radix Wutou, aconite)
huā jiāo (花椒 Zanthoxyli Pericarpium, zanthoxylum)
fù zǐ (附子 Aconiti Radix Lateralis Praeparata, aconite)
gān jiāng (干姜 Zingiberis Rhizoma, dried ginger)
chì shí zhī (赤石脂 Halloysitum Rubrum, halloysite)
Plus:
rén shēn (人参 Ginseng Radix, ginseng)

guì zhī (桂枝 Cinnamomi Ramulus, cinnamon twig)
dāng guī (当归 Angelicae Sinensis Radix, Chinese angelica)
chì sháo (赤芍 Paeoniae Radix Rubra, red peony)
zhì gān cǎo (炙甘草 Glycyrrhizae Radix cum Liquido Fricta, mix-fried licorice)

寒凝血瘀

气为阳，血为阴，阳主动，阴主静，阳气推动而血行，阳气衰而血泣。正如《素问•调经论》所云："血气者，喜温而恶寒，寒则泣而不能流，温则消而去之。"心主血脉，血能正常营运，全赖心阳推动，才能循环无端，周流不息。心阳虚衰，寒从中生，寒主凝滞可使血泣，阳失推动可使血运迟慢，均可导致寒凝血瘀之病机。《医理真传•阳虚症问答》云："心者，气之帅也，心阳得补，而肺气更旺，"这表明肺气盛衰与心阳密切相关。心阳虚衰，肺气受损，胸中阳气不振，气血凝滞胸中，窒塞胸气，发为胸痹。常见胸满喘促，短气不利，胸背引痛，气结咳唾等症。病机的重点是心肺阳气虚衰，而不是痰浊壅盛，治疗宜用补法，温通心阳，散结开痹。方选《金匮要略》人参汤（人参、干姜、白术、甘草）加桂枝、杏仁、桔梗、枳实、橘皮，温脾暖心，补益心阳而收散结开痹之功。若心阳虚衰，寒凝心体血脉，血行迟涩而瘀塞，则为心痛。寒凝血瘀较轻，则为心胸刺痛、后背引痛、反复发作、喜温恶凉。治宜温阳益气，活血化瘀。方用《妇人良方》参附汤加桂枝、当归、川芎、丹参、郁金、甘草。寒凝血瘀较重，心脉痹阻深重，则为心中剧痛暴作、遇寒加重、得温痛减、心痛彻背、背痛彻心、手足冷逆、面唇青紫晦暗、爪甲紫暗、舌质晦暗、舌质尖边有瘀斑瘀点、舌下络脉显露、脉来或促或结或代、或微细欲绝。治宜温阳活血，逐寒止痛。方用《金匮要略》乌头赤石脂丸（乌头、蜀椒、附子、干姜、赤石脂）加人参、桂枝、当归、赤芍、炙甘草。

Literature Review of Congealing Cold with Blood Stasis

📖 *Jīn Guì Yào Lüe* ("Essential Prescriptions of the Golden Coffer"), "Chapter on Disorders of Chest Impediment, Heart Pain, and Shortness of Breath"

"When taking the pulse, one should pay attention to whether it is excessive or deficient. If the yáng pulse is faint and the yīn pulse is stringlike, it indicates chest impediment and pain. The reason for this is found in the extreme state of vacuity. We know that yáng vacuity is located in the upper burner and the condition of chest impediment with heart pain causes a stringlike yīn pulse."

When considering the above-mentioned "faint yáng pulse" together with "we know that yáng vacuity is located in the upper burner," it becomes clear that this refers to an insufficiency of yáng qì in the heart and lungs. When yáng is vacuous and yīn is exuberant, they block the clear area in the center of the chest and prevent yáng qì from moving freely. The static qì and blood cannot move freely, causing pain. This gives rise to chest impediment pain.

📖 *Lèi Zhèng Zhì Cái* ("Systematized Patterns with Clear-Cut Treatments"), "Chest Impediment"

> "In chest impediment, chest yáng is debilitated and unable to move. Over time, yīn overwhelms the position of yáng and causes impediment and binding. This pathocondition is marked by chest fullness, panting, shortness of breath, and inhibited breathing, with pain stretching to the heart and chest. Because yáng qì is constrained in the chest, turbid yīn ascends counterflow to obstruct the upbearing and downbearing of yáng. In severe cases, it causes qì binding with cough, spitting, and chest pain stretching through to the back."

Yáng debility in the chest points to debility of heart yáng; this explains why yáng vacuity can lead to chest impediment with heart pain.

📖 *Zhū Bìng Yuán Hòu Lùn* ("The Origin and Indicators of Disease"), "On Heart Pain"

> "The heart is ascribed to fire and is the confluence of yáng. [Its channel is the] hand lesser yīn channel. If all the yáng qì is vacuous, qì will counterflow in the lesser yīn channel. This is called yáng vacuity yīn reversal and also causes heart pain."

This quotation points out that heart yáng vacuity with obstruction of the heart channel can lead to chest pain.

📖 *Bǐ Huā Yī Jìng* ("*Bǐ Huā* Medical Mirror"), "Heart Section"

> "Heart cold invariably presents with a slow pulse in the left inch position and forms a pathocondition of fulminant pain. The fulminant pain is related to incessant cold limbs and cold qì."

When heart yáng is vacuous, it is unable to warm and move the blood in the vessels. The heart governs the left inch pulse, which arrives slowly and moderately. Obstruction in the heart vessels causes chest pain. When the yáng qì in the blood vessels fails to reach the four limbs, the limbs will be cold.

📖 *Yī Biǎn* ("Signboard on Medicine"), "Heart Pain"

> "The heart is the monarch. It is righteous and must not contract evil. If evil damages [the heart] viscus and causes pain, it is called true heart pain. This pathocondition is marked by sudden great pain, grinding of the

teeth and clenched jaw, cold qì, incessant sweating, a black face, green-blue extremities past the joints that are cold as ice, and a morning onset resulting in death in the evening, or an evening onset resulting in death in the morning. It cannot be treated."

This quotation points out that devitalized heart yáng causes congealing cold and blood stasis that obstructs the heart vessels. This is the most important pathomechanism in chest impediment and heart pain.

文献评述

《金匮要略•胸痹心痛短气病篇》说："夫脉当取太过不及，阳微阴弦，即胸痹而痛。所以然者，责其极虚也。今阳虚知在上焦，所以胸痹心痛者，以其阴弦故也。"其中脉来"阳微"，结合"阳虚知在上焦"，联系起来，可知是心肺阳气不足。阳虚阴盛，闭塞胸中清旷之区，则阳气不通，气血瘀滞，不通则痛，而为胸痹疼痛。

《类证治裁•胸痹》说："胸痹，胸中阳微不运，久则阴乘阳位而为痹结也。其症胸满喘息，短气不利，痛引心背，由胸中阳气不舒，浊阴得以上逆，而阻其升降。甚则气结咳唾，胸痛彻背"。胸中阳微是指心阳虚衰，阐明心阳虚可致胸痹心痛。

《诸病源候论•心痛论》说："心为火，与诸阳会合，而手少阴心之经也。若诸阳气虚，少阴之经气逆，谓之阳虚阴厥，亦令心痛。"指出心阳虚，痹阻心脉，可致胸痛。

《笔花医镜•心部》说："心之寒，脉左寸必迟，其症为暴痛。暴痛者，肢冷气冷，绵绵不休。"心阳虚，不能温通血脉，故主心的左寸脉来迟缓；心脉痹阻而胸痛；阳气血脉不达四肢而肢冷。

《医碥•心痛》说："心为君主，义不受邪，若邪伤其藏而痛者，谓之真心痛。其症卒然大痛，咬牙噤口气冷，汗出不休，面黑，手足青过节，冷如冰，旦发夕死，夕发旦死，不治。"指出心阳不振，寒凝血瘀，心脉阻塞，是形成胸痹、心痛的重要病机。

Summary of Congealing Cold and Blood Stasis

1.   Damage to the Lung Qì
   Chest impediment, chest fullness with hasty panting, short and inhibited breathing, pain stretching through the chest and back, qì binding with cough and spitting
2.   Cold Congealing the Heart Vessels
   Mild patterns: Repeated attacks of stabbing pain in the heart and chest that are followed by pain stretching to the back, liking for warmth, and aversion to coolness

> *Severe patterns*: Sudden attacks of intense pain that are aggravated by exposure to cold and relieved by warmth, with heart pain stretching through to the back or back pain stretching through to the heart, counterflow cold of the limbs, blue-green or purple face and lips, dark purple nails, a dark tongue body with stasis macules and stasis speckles, exposed sublingual network vessels, and a pulse that is skipping, bound, intermittent, or faint and fine verging on expiry

寒凝血瘀

肺气受损 —— 胸痹，胸满喘促，短气不利，胸背引痛，气结咳唾。
寒凝心脉

　　轻证 —— 心胸刺痛、后背引痛、反复发作、喜温恶凉。

　　重证 —— 剧痛暴作、遇寒加重、得温痛减、心痛彻背、背痛彻心、手足冷逆、面唇青紫、爪甲紫暗、舌质晦暗、瘀斑瘀点、舌下络脉显露,脉来或促或结或代、或微细欲绝。

9.3 Insecurity of Heart Yáng

Sweat is the humor associated with the heart. Under normal physiological conditions, heart yáng is able to propel the fluids out of the skin as sweat while simultaneously containing the fluids to avoid excessive sweating. If heart yáng is vacuous, the body's external defense is insecure and unable to contain the fluids; thus, persistent leaking sweat and loose interstices result. This can lead to habitual spontaneous sweating, cold sweating and aversion to wind, and repeated common colds. It should be treated by supplementing heart yáng, and by securing the exterior and checking sweating. For a formula, use Cinnamon Twig and Aconite Decoction (*guì zhī fù zǐ tāng*) from the *Shāng Hán Lùn* ("On Cold Damage"), with the addition of astragalus.

Cinnamon Twig and Aconite Decoction (桂枝附子汤 *guì zhī fù zǐ tāng*)
guì zhī (桂枝 Cinnamomi Ramulus, cinnamon twig)
sháo yào (芍药 Paeoniae Radix, peony)
shēng jiāng (生姜 Zingiberis Rhizoma Recens, fresh ginger)
dà zǎo (大枣 Jujubae Fructus, jujube)
fù zǐ (附子 Aconiti Radix Lateralis Praeparata, aconite)
gān cǎo (甘草 Glycyrrhizae Radix, licorice)
Plus:
huáng qí (黄芪 Astragali Radix, astragalus)

心阳不固

汗为心液，正常生理状态下，心阳既可推动津液从皮肤外出而为汗，同时也能统摄津液，防止汗出过多。如果心阳虚，卫外不固，不能统摄津液，汗漏不止，肌腠疏松，则可引起经常自汗，汗冷怕风，反复感冒等症。治宜补益心阳，固表止汗。方用《伤寒论》<u>桂枝加附子汤</u>（桂枝、芍药、生姜、大枣、附子、甘草）加黄芪。

Literature Review of Insecurity of Heart Yáng

📖 *Jǐng Yuè Quán Shū* ("Jǐng-Yuè's Complete Compendium"), "Schema of Miscellaneous Patterns," "Sweating Patterns"

"It is stated in the appendix to Dān-Xī, 'What the heart stores on the inside is blood, what it distributes to the outside is sweat.' Given the fact that sweat is the humor of the heart, there are no patterns of spontaneous sweating that are not caused by a vacuity of the heart or kidney. The reason for this is that when yīn is vacuous, yáng will invariably encroach, giving rise to heat effusion and spontaneous sweating. When yáng is vacuous, yīn will invariably overwhelm it, giving rise to reversal and spontaneous sweating. Both circumstances are caused by a one-sided prevalence of yīn or yáng."

This quotation emphasizes the close relationship between sweating and the yáng qì of the heart. When yáng is vacuous and yīn is exuberant, yáng qì is unable to defend and secure the outer body; thus, one sees counterflow cold in the four limbs and spontaneous sweating. Yáng vacuity includes heart yáng vacuity; if heart qì is unable to perform its containing function in the outer body, spontaneous sweating results.

📖 *Zá Bìng Yuán Liú Xī Zhú* ("Incisive Light on the Source of Miscellaneous Disease"), "The Source of Sweating"

"Sweating is a heart vacuity disorder. Sweat is the humor of the heart. Thus, when it is pathological, its source always is associated with the heart, even though there can be other factors involved. Although the kidney governs the five humors, if heart yáng is vacuous and unable to secure the outer defense, external damage and spontaneous sweating arise. …Qì vacuity and yáng weakness invariably manifest in a fatigued body and spontaneous sweating."

Sweat is the humor of the heart. When heart yáng is vacuous and unable to secure the outer defense, it is likely to result in spontaneous sweating.

文献评述

《景岳全书•杂证谟•汗证》说："丹溪附录曰：心之所藏在内者
为血，发外者为汗。盖汗乃心之液，而自汗之证未有不由心肾之虚
而得之者。故阴虚阳必凑，发热而自汗；阳虚阴必乘，发厥而自
汗，皆阴阳偏胜所致也。"指出汗出与心的阳气有密切的关系，阳虚
阴盛，阳气不能卫外为固，则四肢逆冷而汗自出。阳虚自然包含心
阳虚在内，心气不能外摄，故而自汗。

《杂病源流犀烛•诸汗源流》说："诸汗，心虚病也。汗者，心之
液，故其为病，虽有别因，其源总属于心。然肾又主五液，心阳虚
不能卫外而为固，则外伤而自汗。…气虚而阳弱者，必体倦而自
汗。"汗为心液，心阳虚不能卫外而固，则易引起自汗。

Summary of Insecurity of Heart Yáng

1. Insecurity of Heart Yáng
    Habitual sweating, cold sweating and aversion to wind, repeated
    common colds

心阳不固

心阳不固 —— 经常汗出，汗冷怕风，反复感冒。

9.4 Water Collection and Liquid Obstruction

It is generally assumed that irregularities in the metabolism of the bodily
fluids are predominantly related to three viscera: the lung, spleen, and
kidney. Thus, it is said that "phlegm caused by vacuity detriment is
never far from an insufficiency of the three channels: spleen, lung, and
kidney," (*Bù Jū Jí* ("Nonlimitation Collection"), "Brief Summary of
Phlegm Patterns"). The heart is thought to be affected more rarely.
Nonetheless, the heart also participates in the process of fluid metabolism.

The heart governs the blood and vessels. A large amount of fluid is
contained in the blood; when heart yáng moves the blood throughout the
entire body, it also sprinkles fluids throughout the body. When heart
yáng is devitalized and fails to warm and move, qì and blood fail to move.
This causes non-distribution of water and liquids, which leads to water
collection and liquid obstruction. Rheum forms and then transforms into
phlegm, which amasses and accumulates to cause various problems.

Alternatively, when spleen and kidney yáng are vacuous, water and
dampness spill over and water qì ascends counterflow to intimidate heart

yáng. If heart yáng is debilitated and unable to distribute and dissipate yīn, the pathomechanism of water qì intimidating the heart arises.

When water collects below the heart, it causes heart stirring and heart palpitations. The qì dynamic becomes depressed, causing counterflow fullness below the heart. This affects the lung's ability to govern breathing, causing shortness of breath. Water may ascend to invade the location of clear yáng, causing dizziness. It may also descend to influence bladder qì transformation, resulting in inhibited urination. These conditions should be treated by warming and supplementing heart yáng while transforming qì and moving water. For a formula, use Poria, Cinnamon Twig, White Atractylodes, and Licorice Decoction (*líng guì zhú gān tāng*) in combination with Poria Five Powder (*wǔ líng sǎn*). Both these formulas are from the *Jīn Guì Yào Lüè* ("Essential Prescriptions of the Golden Coffer").

Poria, Cinnamon Twig, White Atractylodes, and Licorice Decoction (苓桂朮甘汤 *líng guì zhú gān tāng*)

guì zhī (桂枝 Cinnamomi Ramulus, cinnamon twig)
fú líng (茯苓 Poria, poria)
bái zhú (白朮 Atractylodis Macrocephalae Rhizoma, white atractylodes)
gān cǎo (甘草 Glycyrrhizae Radix, licorice)

Poria Five Powder (五苓散 *wǔ líng sǎn*)

guì zhī (桂枝 Cinnamomi Ramulus, cinnamon twig)
fú líng (茯苓 Poria, poria)
zé xiè (泽泻 Alismatis Rhizoma, alisma)
bái zhú (白朮 Atractylodis Macrocephalae Rhizoma, white atractylodes)
zhū líng (猪苓 Polyporus, polyporus)

If heart yáng is vacuous and therefore unable to transform qì and move water, water collects in the chest and forms phlegm turbidity. This can lead to the pathomechanism of cold phlegm and blood stasis binding together, which in turn leads to chest impediment. Cold phlegm obstructing the heart vessels can manifest as stifling oppression, distention, and pain in the heart and chest, heart palpitations, and shortness of breath.

When phlegm stasis obstructs chest yáng, it causes manifestations of widespread yīn cold, such as pain stretching through the chest and back, panting, coughing and spitting, a pale and swollen tongue with thick slimy fur, and a stringlike and slippery pulse. This should be treated by warming and supplementing heart yáng while sweeping phlegm and transforming stasis. For a formula, use a combination of the *Jīn Guì Yào*

Lüe ("Essential Prescriptions of the Golden Coffer") formulas Ginseng Decoction (*rén shēn tāng*) and Poria, Cinnamon Twig, White Atractylodes, and Licorice Decoction (*líng guì zhú gān tāng*), with the addition of Chinese chive, pinellia, salvia, chuanxiong, and dalbergia.

Ginseng Decoction (人参汤 *rén shēn tāng*)
rén shēn (人参 Ginseng Radix, ginseng)
gān jiāng (干姜 Zingiberis Rhizoma, dried ginger)
bái zhú (白朮 Atractylodis Macrocephalae Rhizoma, white atractylodes)
gān cǎo (甘草 Glycyrrhizae Radix, licorice)

Poria, Cinnamon Twig, White Atractylodes, and Licorice Decoction (苓桂朮甘汤 *líng guì zhú gān tāng*)
guì zhī (桂枝 Cinnamomi Ramulus, cinnamon twig)
fú líng (茯苓 Poria, poria)
bái zhú (白朮 Atractylodis Macrocephalae Rhizoma, white atractylodes)
gān cǎo (甘草 Glycyrrhizae Radix, licorice)
Plus:
xiè bái (薤白 Allii Macrostemonis Bulbus, Chinese chive)
bàn xià (半夏 Pinelliae Rhizoma, pinellia)
dān shēn (丹参 Salviae Miltiorrhizae Radix, salvia)
chuān xiōng (川芎 Chuanxiong Rhizoma, chuanxiong)
jiàng xiāng (降香 Dalbergiae Odiferae Lignum, dalbergia)

The lesser yīn channel passes through the throat and clasps the root of the tongue. If heart yáng is debilitated, yáng qì loses its ability to warm and move; thus it cannot warm and free the vessels of the lesser yīn channel. The movement of water and liquid is thus inhibited, which forms cold phlegm. This causes binding in the throat and stasis in the blood vessels. Alternatively, if constitutional vacuity of heart yáng is compounded by externally contracted cold evil, the cold congeals the liquids and blood in the throat. Both of these situations can manifest with diffuse swelling and pain in the throat, a dark red color in the throat, cough and vomiting of phlegm-drool, a hoarse voice, and a pale tongue with white fur. This condition should be treated by supplementing heart yáng while transforming phlegm and opening binds. For a formula, use Pinellia powder and decoction (*bàn xià sǎn jí tāng*) from the *Shāng Hán Lùn* ("On Cold Damage"), with the addition of curcuma, red peony, dalbergia, and platycodon.

> ## Pinellia powder and decoction (半夏散及汤 *bàn xià sǎn jí tāng*)
>
> *guì zhī* (桂枝 Cinnamomi Ramulus, cinnamon twig)
> *bàn xià* (半夏 Pinelliae Rhizoma, pinellia)
> *zhì gān cǎo* (炙甘草 Glycyrrhizae Radix cum Liquido Fricta, mix-fried licorice)
> Plus:
> *yù jīn* (郁金 Curcumae Radix, curcuma)
> *chì sháo* (赤芍 Paeoniae Radix Rubra, red peony)
> *jiàng xiāng* (降香 Dalbergiae Odiferae Lignum, dalbergia)
> *jié gěng* (桔梗 Platycodonis Radix, platycodon)

The pinellia in this formula transforms phlegm and dissipates binds. This shows that the sore throat in this case is caused by congealing liquid and blood from cold depressing in the throat. Cinnamon twig warms and frees heart yáng; this shows that the throat pain is caused by heart yáng debility preventing qì from transforming fluids. This ultimately causes collection and obstruction of water and liquids.

水停津阻

一般认为，水液代谢失调，主要与肺脾肾三脏有关。故有"虚损之痰，总不离脾肺肾三经之不足也"（《不居集•痰证扼要》）之说，较少涉及于心。实际上心亦参加水液代谢的过程。心主血脉，血中含有大量津液，心阳推动血液运行全身时，亦将津液洒布全身。如心阳不振，温运失职，在伴随气血失运的同时，亦常发生水津失布，水停津阻，生饮化痰，蓄积为患的病机。或脾肾阳虚，水湿泛溢，水气上逆，凌侮心阳，此时正值心阳已衰不能布散阴弥，又可发生水气凌心的病机。水停心下，心动不安而心悸；气机郁滞而心下逆满；影响肺主呼吸而气短；向上犯及清阳之位而眩晕；向下影响膀胱气化而小便不利。治宜温补心阳，化气行水。方用《金匮要略》苓桂术甘汤（桂枝、茯苓、白术、甘草）合五苓散（桂枝、茯苓、泽泻、白术、猪苓）。

若心阳虚弱，不能充分化气行水，水停胸中，化生痰浊，可致寒痰血瘀互结的病机，引起胸痹。寒痰痹阻心脉可见心胸憋闷胀痛、心悸气短；痰瘀阻碍胸阳，一派阴寒弥漫之象，则胸背引痛、喘息咳唾、舌淡胖、苔厚腻、脉弦滑。治宜温补心阳，豁痰化瘀。方用《金匮要略》人参汤合苓桂术甘汤加薤白、半夏、丹参、川芎、降香。

少阴经脉，循喉咙，挟舌本，若心阳虚衰，阳气失于温煦、推动，不能温通少阴经脉，水津运行不利，化为寒痰，胶结咽喉，瘀滞血脉，或心阳素虚又外感寒邪，寒凝津血于咽喉，均可见咽喉漫肿疼痛、喉间暗红、咳吐痰涎、声音嘶哑、舌淡苔白等症。治宜补益心阳，化痰开结。方用《伤寒论》<u>半夏散及汤</u>（桂枝、半夏、炙甘草）加郁金、赤芍、降香、桔梗。方中半夏化痰散结，可知此咽痛为寒郁咽喉，津血凝滞。桂枝温通心阳，可知此类咽喉疼痛，是由心阳虚衰，气不化津，水津停阻所致。

Literature Review of Water Collection and Liquid Obstruction

📖 *Jīn Guì Yào Lüè* ("Essential Prescriptions of the Golden Coffer"), "Chapter on Phlegm-Rheum Cough Diseases"

> "Water in the heart causes hardness and pounding below the heart, shortness of breath, aversion to water, and no desire to drink."

This quotation points out that damage to heart yáng can cause yáng qì to fail to move, leading to the collection of water below the heart. This results in hard glomus below the heart, palpitations below the heart, and no thought of drinking water. Heart yáng vacuity can progress to cause lung qì weakness; this prevents the lung from being in charge of breathing, leading to shortness of breath.

📖 *Shāng Hán Míng Lǐ Lùn* ("The Clear Rationale of Cold Damage"), "Palpitations"

> "The collection of rheum is caused by water collecting below the heart. The heart belongs to fire and is averse to water. When water collects internally, the heart itself is disquieted, leading to palpitations."

This quotation analyzes in more detail how heart yáng vacuity results in rheum collecting below the heart. Rheum collecting below the heart causes heart stirring and heart palpitations.

📖 *Xuè Zhèng Lùn* ("Treatise on Blood Patterns"), "On the Pathomechanisms of the Bowels and Viscera"

> "When water-rheum restrains fire, the heart has stirring palpitations."

This quotation points out that when water qì invades the heart, heart palpitations may result.

📖 *Jīn Guì Yào Lüè* ("Essential Prescriptions of the Golden Coffer"), "Chapter on the Diseases of Chest Impediment, Heart Pain, and Shortness of Breath"

> "The disease of chest impediment manifests as panting, coughing and spitting, chest and back pain, and shortness of breath."

The *Yī Zōng Jīn Jiàn* ("The Golden Mirror of Orthodox Medicine") comments on the meaning of this quotation:

> "Once yáng qì becomes vacuous, all cold yīn evils overwhelm. This causes qì impediment and stoppage in the chest and back. In mild cases, the patient has fullness; in severe cases, there is pain. Panting, coughing and spitting, and shortness of breath are inevitable [symptoms of this condition]."

When chest impediment and chest pain occur simultaneously and one observes the symptoms of panting, coughing and spitting, and shortness of breath, it means that heart yáng vacuity, cold phlegm, and blood stasis are all present together.

📖 *Shāng Hán Lùn* ("On Cold Damage"), "Lesser Yīn Diseases: Pulses, Patterns and Treatments"

> "When in lesser yīn disease, [there is] soreness in the throat, Pinellia Powder and Decoction governs."

📖 The *Shāng Hán Guàn Zhū Jí* ("A Collected String of Pearls on Cold Damage") expounds on the meaning of this quotation:

> "Lesser yīn throat pain… [results] when lesser yīn cold evil is depressed and gathers in the throat, unable to either exit or enter."

Lesser yīn is associated with the heart and kidney. When kidney yáng is vacuous, it is unable to warm heart yáng. This can cause devitalized heart yáng and a failure of qì to transform liquids. If external evils invade and ascend along the lesser yīn channel to invade the throat, cold phlegm congealing in the throat causes diffuse swelling and soreness in the throat.

文献评述

《金匮要略•痰饮咳嗽病篇》说："水在心，心下坚筑，短气，恶水不欲饮。"指出心阳受损，阳气失运，水停心下，可致心下痞硬，心下悸动，不思饮水；心阳虚，进而引起肺气弱，不司呼吸，可致短气。

《伤寒明理论•悸》说："其停饮者，由水停心下，心为火而恶水，水既内停，心自不安，则为悸也。"进一步阐述心阳虚，心下停饮，心动不安，而为心悸。

《血证论•脏腑病机论》说："水饮克火，心亦动悸。"亦指出水气犯心，可致心悸。

《金匮要略•胸痹心痛短气病篇》说："胸痹之病，喘息咳唾，胸背痛，短气。"《医宗金鉴》注解其义时说："阳气一虚，诸寒阴邪得以乘之，则胸背之气痹而不通，轻则病满，重者病痛，理之必然也。喘息咳唾，短气证之必有也。"在胸痹胸痛的同时，见喘息咳唾之症，是心阳虚，寒痰与血瘀共存所致。

《伤寒论•辨少阴病脉证并治》"少阴病，咽中痛，半夏散及汤主之。"《伤寒贯珠集》在阐述其义时说："少阴咽痛，…盖少阴寒邪郁聚咽嗌之间，既不得出，复不得入。"少阴属心肾，肾阳虚不能温暖心阳，可致心阳不振，气不化津，沿少阴经脉上犯于咽喉，加之寒邪外犯，寒痰凝滞咽喉，则为咽喉漫肿疼痛。

Summary of Water Collection and Liquid Obstruction
1. **Water Qì Intimidating the Heart** Heart palpitations, counterflow fullness below the heart, shortness of breath, dizziness, inhibited urination 2. **Cold Phlegm Congealing in the Heart** Stifling oppression, distention, and pain in the heart and chest; pain stretching through the chest and back; panting, coughing, and spitting; heart palpitations with shortness of breath; pale and enlarged tongue with thick and slimy fur; string-like and slippery pulse 3. **Cold Congealing in the Throat** Diffuse swelling and soreness in the throat, dark and red coloration in the throat, coughing and spitting of phlegm-drool, hoarse voice, pale tongue with white fur
水停津阻
水气凌心 —— 心悸，心下逆满，气短，眩晕，小便不利。 寒痰凝心 —— 心胸憋闷胀痛、胸背引痛、喘息咳唾、心悸气短、舌淡胖、苔厚腻、脉弦滑 寒凝咽喉 —— 咽喉漫肿疼痛、喉间暗红、咳吐痰涎、声音嘶哑、舌淡苔白。

Heart yáng debility may lead to pathological changes such as dual vacuity of heart yīn and heart yáng, heart-spleen yáng vacuity, heart-lung yáng vacuity, or heart-kidney yáng vacuity.

Dual Vacuity of Yīn and Yáng in the Heart

In heart yáng insufficiency, yáng vacuity leaves yīn with nothing to transform; over time, the yáng detriment affects yīn. This can cause heart yīn insufficiency and form the pathomechanism of dual vacuity of heart yīn and yáng. It manifests with chest oppression and heart pain, physical cold and cold limbs, heat vexation in the five hearts, and a red bare smooth tongue. This pathocondition is a cold-heat complex.

Heart-Spleen Yáng Vacuity

The heart is ascribed to fire and the spleen and stomach are ascribed to earth. According to the law of engenderment among the five phases, heart fire has the function of assisting the spleen by warming earth. When heart yáng is vacuous, fire is unable to warm earth; this can lead to vacuity cold in the spleen and stomach. This manifests as chest pain, chest oppression, and a somber face and dark tongue; in addition, there may be dull pain in the stomach and stomach duct that likes warmth and pressure.

Heart-Lung Yáng Vacuity

The heart and lung are both located in the upper burner. Lung qì passes through the heart vessels to move blood. Prolonged heart yáng debility invariably results in depletion of yáng qì in the lung, causing the pathomechanism of heart-lung yáng vacuity. This manifests as heart palpitations and chest pain, physical cold and cold in the limbs, as well as panting, coughing, and spitting.

Heart-Kidney Yáng Vacuity

The heart above interacts with the kidney below; water and fire thus help each other. When heart yáng is debilitated, it is unable to warm kidney yáng below. This can lead to kidney water (a type of water swelling) with congealing cold and water qì intimidating the heart. This process is involved in the pathomechanism of heart-kidney yáng vacuity. Patients will first present with heart palpitations and shortness of breath, followed by severe water swelling in the lower extremities and cold aching lumbus and knees.

When heart yáng has been critically damaged or when heart yáng vacuity occurs in recurrent attacks of gradually increasing severity, yáng becomes extremely vacuous and ancestral qì is greatly discharged. This can give rise to the pathomechanism of fulminant desertion of heart yáng.

心的阴阳两虚：心阳不足，阳虚则阴无以化，继而阳损及阴，可至心阴不足，形成心的阴阳两虚的病机。既有胸闷心痛，形寒肢冷，又有五心烦热，舌红光滑之症，为寒热错杂之证。

心脾阳虚：心属火，脾胃属土，按照五行相生规律，心火有助脾暖土的功能。心阳虚，火不暖土，可引起脾胃虚寒。既见胸痛胸闷，面舌晦暗，又可见胃脘隐痛，喜温喜按等症。

心肺阳虚：心肺同居上焦，肺气贯心脉行血，当心阳虚衰时，久之必导致肺的阳气亏损，引起心肺阳虚的病机。既见心悸胸痛，形寒肢冷，又见喘息咳唾等症。

心肾阳虚：心肾上下相交，水火既济，心阳虚衰，不能下温肾阳，可致肾水寒凝和水气凌心，引起心肾阳虚的病机。病人先有心悸气短，而后出现水肿下肢尤甚，腰膝酸冷等症。

心阳虚反复发作，逐渐加剧，或心阳受到严重损伤，阳虚至极，宗气大泄，可形成心阳暴脱的病机。

Chapter Ten

Heart Blood Vacuity

In the *Huáng Dì Nèi Jīng* ("The Yellow Emperor's Inner Canon"), we find only a general discussion of blood vacuity. The term "heart blood vacuity" is not mentioned specifically. Heart vacuity patterns are mentioned in discussions on pathomechanisms of the bowels and viscera in the texts *Zhū Bìng Yuán Hòu Lùn* ("The Origin and Indicators of Disease"), the *Qiān Jīn Yào Fāng* ("A Thousand Gold Pieces Prescriptions"), and the *Shèng Jì Zǒng Lù* ("Sages' Salvation Records"). However, these texts tend to mention "blood and qì debility and shortage" together.

The *Jì Shēng Fāng* ("Formulas for Saving Lives") introduces the concept of "heart blood insufficiency" on its own. This is the earliest and most precise exposition of the causes of heart blood vacuity and the pathomechanisms involved. For example, the chapter, "Entry on Fright Palpitations, Fearful Throbbing, and Forgetfulness" states, "Fearful throbbing indicates an insufficiency of heart blood. The heart governs blood, yet blood also governs the heart. The heart is the monarch of the physical body. Thus, when blood is plentiful, the heart-monarch is naturally quiet. It is mostly because of a desire for wealth and rank and shunning of poverty, or an excessive longing for one's desires or dissatisfaction with one's circumstances, that the true blood is made vacuous and the heart-emperor loses support. This gradually gives rise to fearful throbbing."

Following this, the texts *Yī Xué Rù Mén* ("The Gateway to Medicine"), *Zá Bìng Yuán Liú Xī Zhú* ("Incisive Light on the Source of Miscellaneous Disease"), *Zhèng Zhì Zhǔn Shéng* ("The Level-Line of Pattern Identification and Treatment"), and *Zhèng Zhì Huì Bǔ* ("A Supplement to Patterns and Treatment") employ the expression "singular vacuity of heart blood."

The specific term "heart blood vacuity" is not used until the *Zhèng Yīn Mài Zhì* ("Pathoconditions: Causes, Pulses, and Treatments"). Here, in the section titled "Internal Damage Sleeplessness," it is stated, "The pathocondition of heart blood vacuity sleeplessness manifests with heart vexation and agitation, awakening with fright during the night, dryness of the mouth and tongue, and vexing heat in the five hearts. This is a pathocondition of heart blood insufficiency with excessively effulgent heart fire." Following this text, descriptions of the pathomechanisms of heart blood vacuity have become increasingly complete and have been used extensively to explain many types of disease patterns.

Heart blood vacuity has a variety of causes. It is often caused by excessive thought and preoccupation wearing on yīn-blood. Heart blood vacuity may also result from impaired movement of the spleen-stomach with insufficient transformation and engenderment. Another possible cause is excessive blood loss that reduces heart blood. Additional causes include enduring warm-heat lodged in the body that damages liquids and wears on the blood, as well as damage to heart qì that subsequently affects the blood. Finally, weak health due to enduring illness or lack of treatment or inappropriate treatment may also result in heart blood vacuity.

The blood is the material foundation for the activities of the heart spirit; thus, the pathomechanisms of heart blood vacuity primarily present with irregularities of the heart spirit. The vessels are the house of the blood, so insufficiency of heart blood may manifest in blood vessels that are deprived of nourishment. Additionally, in insufficiency of heart blood, blood vacuity causes qì to be deprived of its foundation; this may result in the pathomechanism of blood vacuity with floating yáng.

心血虚

《黄帝内经》只有血虚的笼统论述，尚未提到心血虚的名称。《诸病源候论》、《千金要方》、《圣济总录》讨论脏腑病机，提到心的虚证时，往往多是"血气衰少"并提。《济生方》中开始有"心血不足"的提法，如该书《惊悸怔忡健忘门》指出："夫怔忡者，此心血不足也。盖心主于血，血乃心之主，心乃形之君，血富则心君自安矣。多因汲汲富贵，戚戚贫贱，又思所爱，触事不意，真血虚耗，心帝失辅，渐成怔忡。"这是对心血虚病因病机最早、最精辟的论述。其后《医学入门》、《杂病源流犀烛》、《证治准绳》、《证治汇补》则采用"心血一虚"等提法。直到《症因脉治》才最准确地使用"心血虚"的名称。是书《内伤不得卧》中说："心血虚不得卧之症，心烦躁乱，夜卧惊起，口燥舌干，五心烦热，此心血不足，心火太旺之症也。"至此之后，有关心血虚病机的论述更加完善，广泛用于阐述各种病证。

心血虚，多由思虑过度，暗耗阴血；或脾胃失运，生化不足；或失血过多，心血减少；或温热久恋，伤津耗血；或心气先伤，由气及血；或久病体弱，失治误治所致。由于血液是心神活动的物质基础，故心血虚的病机主要表现为心神失调。其次，脉为血之府，当心血不足时，亦可见到血脉失养的病机。此外，心血不足，血虚气无所依，可致血虚阳浮的病机。

10.1   Heart Spirit Irregularities

The *Bǐ Huā Yī Jìng* ("*Bǐ Huā* Medical Mirror"), "Section on the Heart," states, "The body of the heart is ascribed to fire. It is located in the south and its color manifests as red. ...It is only when it receives the nourishment of blood that it is able to move intelligence and employ talent and wisdom."

This quotation points out that the heart governs the blood and the blood nourishes the spirit. The heart spirit depends on the blood to guard the essence-spirit internally and to quiet the spirit-mind. Thus, the essence-spirit will be abundant, the spirit-light will be clear and bright, and consciousness will be clear. Thoughts will be sensitive and quick, wisdom will be acute and bright, and memory will be faultless. When heart blood is depleted, the heart spirit is deprived of nourishment and the spirit-light is ungoverned. This can result in irregularities of the heart spirit.

Depending on the different manifestations of heart spirit irregularities, the pathomechanisms can be differentiated into three categories: insufficiency of spirit-qì, spirit failing to keep to its abode, and visceral agitation due to blood vacuity.

心神失调

《笔花医镜•心部》云："心体属火，位南方，色现赤...得血以养之，方能运慧思，用才智。"指出心主血，血养神。心神依赖血的供养，精神内守，神志安宁，故乃精神充沛，神明清朗，意识清楚，思维敏捷，智慧聪明，记忆不忘。心血亏损，心神失养，神明无主，则会引起心神失调。根据精神失调表现的不同，其病机变化可分为神气不足、神不守舍和血虚脏躁三个方面。

10.2   Spirit-Qì Insufficiency

When heart blood is insufficient, blood fails to nourish the spirit and the function of the heart to govern the spirit-mind is reduced. The spirit-mind is thus unable to oversee the normal activities of the essence-spirit, thoughts, and consciousness, leading to spirit-qì insufficiency. This

commonly manifests as a pathocondition of devitalized essence-spirit
with lack of concentration, torpid responses, and forgetfulness. It should
be treated by supplementing heart blood and vitalizing the essence-spirit.
For a formula, use Spirit-Nourishing Pill (*yǎng shén wán*) from the *Shèng
Jì Zǒng Lù* ("Sages' Salvation Records"), with the addition of longan
flesh, white peony, and placenta.

Spirit-Nourishing Pill (养神丸 *yǎng shén wán*)

shú dì huáng (熟地黄 Rehmanniae Radix Praeparata, cooked rehmannia)
rén shēn (人参 Ginseng Radix, ginseng)
fú shén (茯神 Poria cum Pini Radice, root poria)
yuǎn zhì (远志 Polygalae Radix, polygala)
shí chāng pú (石菖蒲 Acori Tatarinowii Rhizoma, acorus)
bái zhú (白术 Atractylodis Macrocephalae Rhizoma, white atractylodes)
shān yào (山药 Dioscoreae Rhizoma, dioscorea)
mài dōng (麦冬 Ophiopogonis Radix, ophiopogon)
zhì gān cǎo (炙甘草 Glycyrrhizae Radix cum Liquido Fricta,
    mix-fried licorice)
Plus:
lóng yǎn ròu (龙眼肉 Longan Arillus, longan flesh)
bái sháo (白芍 Paeoniae Radix Alba, white peony)
zǐ hé chē (紫河车 Hominis Placenta, placenta)

神气不足

　　心血不足，血不养神，心主神志的功能活动衰减，不能从事正常
的精神思维意识活动，而致神气不足。常见精神不振，思想不集
中，反应迟钝，健忘遗事等症。治宜补养心血，振奋精神。方用
《圣济总录》养神丸（熟地、人参、茯神、远志、石菖蒲、白术、
山药、麦冬、炙甘草）加圆肉、白芍、紫河车。

Literature Review of Spirit Qì Insufficiency

📖 *Shèng Jì Zǒng Lù* ("Sages' Salvation Records"), "Heart Forgetfulness"

> "The disease of forgetfulness is rooted in the heart. Debility of blood and
> qì leads to clouding and fretting of the essence-spirit, which causes stir-
> ring and derangement of the mind and forgetfulness."

This quotation points out that in heart blood insufficiency, blood fails to
nourish the spirit, resulting in a devitalized essence-spirit and forgetfulness.

📖 *Jì Shēng Fāng* ("Formulas for Saving Lives"), "Entry on Fright Palpitations, Fearful Throbbing, and Forgetfulness"

"Forgetfulness is a constant tendency to forget things. Although the spleen governs thought and reflection, the heart also governs thought. Excessive thinking and preoccupation causes the abode of reflection to lack essence and impairs the spirit palace. This results in forgetfulness."

This quotation points out that thought and preoccupation damage the heart, causing heart blood to be insufficient. The heart spirit is deprived of nourishment and spirit and thought are ungoverned. This can result in forgetfulness.

📖 *Shòu Shì Bǎo Yuán* ("Prolonging Life and Preserving the Origin"), "Forgetfulness"

"Forgetfulness refers to the condition whereby a person suddenly forgets their affairs. Despite great effort of the mind, they cannot recall things. They begin jobs but leave them unfinished, and when speaking, they do not know the beginning or end [of their sentences]. This process is governed by the two channels of the heart and spleen. Thought is governed by the office of the heart as well as by the office of the spleen. Excessive thought and preoccupation damage the heart by wearing and dissipating blood; this causes the spirit to fail to keep to its abode. Damage to the spleen causes stomach qì to be debilitated and exhausted, allowing disease to penetrate more deeply. These two channels [heart and spleen] both govern the person's affairs; thus, sudden forgetfulness can result."

This quotation elaborates on the pathomechanisms of forgetfulness, which involve heart blood debility causing the heart spirit to be ungoverned.

文献评述

《圣济总录•心健忘》说："健忘之病，本属于心，血气衰少，精神昏愦，故志动乱而多忘也。"指出心血不足，血不养神，可致精神不振、健忘遗事。

《济生方•惊悸怔忡健忘门》说："夫健忘者，常常喜忘是也。盖脾主意与思，心亦主思，思虑过度，意舍不精，神宫不职，使人健忘。"指出思虑伤心，心血不足，心神失养，不主神思，可致健忘。

《寿世保元•健忘》云："夫健忘者，陡然而忘其事也。尽心力思量不来，为事有始无终，言谈不知首尾。盖主于心脾二经，心之官则思，脾之官亦主思，由此思虑过度，伤心则血耗散，神不守舍。伤脾则胃气衰惫，而疾愈深。二者皆主人事，则卒然而忘也。"进一步阐明健忘遗事的病机是心血虚衰，心神无主。

10.3   Spirit Failing to Keep to Its Abode

When heart blood is insufficient, it is unable to nourish the heart. The spirit will not be constrained, so spirit qì will fail to keep its composure and will be disquieted. Thus, there will be agitation and stirring of the heart spirit. This results in heart palpitations, fearful throbbing, fright, and fear.

If blood fails to nourish the heart, the heart spirit floats astray. When the spirit fails to keep to its abode, the spirit and the corporeal soul wander outward, causing insomnia and profuse dreaming. This should be treated by supplementing heart blood while quieting the heart and spirit. For a formula, use Heart-Nourishing Decoction (*yǎng xīn tāng*) from the *Gǔ Jīn Yī Tǒng Dà Quán* ("The Complete Compendium of Medical Works, Ancient and Modern").

Heart-Nourishing Decoction (养心丸 *yǎng xīn tāng*)

rén shēn (人参 Ginseng Radix, ginseng)

dāng guī (当归 Angelicae Sinensis Radix, Chinese angelica)

shēng dì huáng (生地黄 Rehmanniae Radix Exsiccata seu Recens, dried/fresh rehmannia)

shú dì huáng (熟地黄 Rehmanniae Radix Praeparata, cooked rehmannia)

fú shén (茯神 Poria cum Pini Radice, root poria)

mài dōng (麦冬 Ophiopogonis Radix, ophiopogon)

wǔ wèi zǐ (五味子 Schisandrae Fructus, schisandra)

zhì gān cǎo (炙甘草 Glycyrrhizae Radix cum Liquido Fricta, mix-fried licorice)

To treat this condition, the formula Spleen-Returning Decoction (*guī pí tāng*) may also be chosen. Spleen-Returning Decoction (*guī pí tāng*) comes from the text *Jì Shēng Fāng* ("Formulas for Saving Lives").

Spleen-Returning Decoction (归脾汤 *guī pí tāng*)

huáng qí (黄芪 Astragali Radix, astragalus)

rén shēn (人参 Ginseng Radix, ginseng)

dāng guī (当归 Angelicae Sinensis Radix, Chinese angelica)

bái zhú (白术 Atractylodis Macrocephalae Rhizoma, white atractylodes)

suān zǎo rén (酸枣仁 Ziziphi Spinosi Semen, spiny jujube)

lóng yǎn ròu (龙眼肉 Longan Arillus, longan flesh)

yuǎn zhì (远志 Polygalae Radix, polygala)

fú líng (茯苓 Poria, poria)

mù xiāng (木香 Aucklandiae Radix, costusroot)

gān cǎo (甘草 Glycyrrhizae Radix, licorice)

神不守舍

心血不足，不能养心，失于敛神，神气失守，不得安宁，心神躁动，则为心悸怔忡，惊恐不安。若血不养心，心神浮越，神不守舍，神魄外游，则为失眠多梦。治宜补养心血，宁心安神。方用《古今医统》养心汤（人参、当归、生地黄、熟地黄、茯神、麦冬、五味子、炙甘草）。也可选用《济生方》归脾汤（黄芪、人参、当归、白术、酸枣仁、圆肉、远志、茯苓、木香、甘草）治疗。

Literature Review of Spirit Failing to Keep its Abode

📖 *Dān Xī Xīn Fǎ* ("Dān-Xī's Heart-Approach"), "Fright Palpitations and Fearful Throbbing"

> "Man is governed by the heart. The heart is nourished by blood. Singular vacuity of heart blood causes spirit qì to fail to keep its composure. This is the origin of fright palpitations."

This quotation describes the pathomechanism through which insufficiency of heart blood causes blood to fail to nourish the spirit. Spirit qì thus fails to keep its composure, resulting in fright palpitations.

📖 *Yī Xué Rù Mén* ("The Gateway to Medicine"), "The Pathoconditions of Fearful Throbbing, Fright Palpitations, and Forgetfulness"

> "The symptoms of fearful throbbing and fright palpitations…are potentially due to fright qì entering the gallbladder. The mother can make the child vacuous, resulting in heart blood insufficiency. Alternatively, when one is exposed to manifold and tedious affairs and engages one's thoughts endlessly, the heart sovereign can become disquiet. This causes the spirit-light to be disquieted, giving rise to the pathoconditions of fearful throbbing and fright palpitations."

This quotation points out that heart blood insufficiency and disquietude of the spirit-light can result in fright palpitations and fearful throbbing.

📖 *Zá Bìng Yuán Liú Xī Zhú* ("Incisive Light on the Source of Miscellaneous Disease"), "The Source of Fearful Throbbing"

> "Fearful throbbing is a disease of heart blood insufficiency. Man is governed by the heart. The heart is governed by blood. Dissipation and collapse of heart blood causes spirit qì to fail to keep its composure. This results in constant emptiness in the heart, discontent, stirring, shaking, and disquietude. This is called fearful throbbing."

This quotation points out that heart blood insufficiency and failure of blood to nourish the spirit can result in heart palpitations and fearful throbbing. This occurs because spirit qì fails to keep its composure, causing stirring, shaking, and instability.

📖 *Xuè Zhèng Lùn* ("Treatise on Blood Patterns"), "On the Pathomechanisms of the Bowels and Viscera"

> "The heart holds the office of monarch, whence the spirit-light emanates. …Blood vacuity causes a disquieted spirit and fearful throbbing. The presence of static blood also causes fearful throbbing."

Blood failing to nourish the heart may result from blood vacuity or static blood obstruction. This causes a disquieted heart spirit, which leads to heart palpitations and fearful throbbing.

📖 *Féng Shì Jǐn Náng Mì Lù* ("Feng's Brocade Bag Secret Record"), "Correlating Formulas and Pulses in Fright Palpitations, Fearful Throbbing, and Forgetfulness"

> "Fearful throbbing refers to throbbing and stirring in the heart and fear as if about to be arrested. The stirring is aggravated by thought and preoccupation. This is all ascribed to blood vacuity."

This quotation points out that insufficiency of heart blood and the subsequent failure of blood to nourish the heart results in heart stirring, heart palpitations, and fearful throbbing.

📖 *Biàn Zhèng Lù* ("Record of Pattern Identification"), "Entry on Fright Palpitation"

> "When the ethereal and corporeal souls are unstable, fright is generated. When the ethereal and corporeal souls are disquieted, palpitations arise. Both of these are related to blood vacuity in the regions of the heart and liver. In cases of blood vacuity, the spirit has no place to return to and the ethereal soul is ungoverned."

This quotation points out that heart blood vacuity and the subsequent failure of blood to nourish the spirit causes the ethereal and corporeal souls to be unstable, generating fright palpitations.

📖 *Jǐng Yuè Quán Shū* ("Jǐng-Yuè's Complete Compendium"), "Schema of Miscellaneous Patterns" and "Sleeplessness"

> "Sleeplessness without the presence of evil is due to an insufficiency of construction qì. Construction governs blood; when blood is vacuous, it is unable to nourish the heart. When the heart is vacuous, the spirit fails to keep to its abode. This can cause symptoms such as fright and jerking or fear, possibly as if one's thoughts are fixated on something. It may also cause profuse and frenetic thoughts without a cause, to the point of sleeplessness all night or alternate sleeping and waking, or disquietude as if caused by ghosts and spirits."

This quotation points out that when heart blood is insufficient, blood fails to nourish the spirit, the spirit fails to keep to its abode, and the ethereal and corporeal souls roam astray. This can result in insomnia and profuse dreaming.

📖 *Zá Bìng Yuán Liú Xī Zhú* ("Incisive Light on the Source of Miscellaneous Disease"), "The Origin of Heart Disease"

> "The heart governs the body and controls the sea of blood. Thus, when heart blood is scanty, the spirit is unstable, sleep is disquieted, and the hundred diseases gather and arise."

The heart governs the blood vessels. When heart blood is vacuous, blood fails to nourish the spirit, and the spirit and ethereal soul are unstable. This can result in insomnia.

📖 *Gǔ Jīn Yī Tǒng Dà Quán* ("The Complete Compendium of Medical Works, Ancient and Modern")

> "The heart is the perch of the spirit. Whenever thought and preoccupation are excessive, heart blood is depleted and the spirit roams to the outside. This causes profuse dreaming."

This quotation describes that an insufficiency of heart blood causes the spirit to roam outside; this gives rise to insomnia and profuse dreaming.

📖 *Zhèng Zhì Huì Bǔ* ("A Supplement to Patterns and Treatment"), "Fright Palpitations and Fearful Throbbing"

> "The disease of bēi dié is marked by glomus blockage in the chest with no desire for food or drink, a constant sense of lack in the heart, and a preference for staying in a dark room or for standing by the door observing people. This sensation reaches the point of being so frightened as to want to disappear from the face of the earth, resembling someone who has lost their mind. This is caused by heart blood insufficiency; treat it with Ginseng Construction-Nourishing Decoction."

This quotation points out that heart blood insufficiency that fails to nourish the spirit can result in derangement of the essence-spirit. This can lead to pathoconditions of burning preoccupation and fear, as well as heart palpitations.

文献评述

　　《丹溪心法·惊悸怔忡》说："人之所主者心，心之所养者血，心血一虚，神气不守，此惊悸之所肇端也。"精辟地阐述了心血不足，血不养神，神气不守而致惊悸的病机。

《医学入门•怔忡惊悸健忘症》说："夫怔忡惊悸之候，…或因惊气入胆，母能令子虚，因而心血为之不足。又或遇事繁冗，思想无穷，则心君亦为之不宁，故神明不安而怔忡惊悸之症作矣。"也指出心血不足，神明不宁，可致惊悸怔忡。

《杂病源流犀烛•怔忡源流》说："怔忡，心血不足病也。人所主者心，心所主者血，心血消亡，神气失守，则心中空虚，怏怏动摇，不得安宁，无时不作，名曰怔忡。"指出心血不足，血不养神，神气失守，动摇不定，可致心悸怔忡。

《血证论•脏腑病机论》说："心者君主之官，神明出焉。…血虚则神不安而怔忡，有瘀血亦怔忡。"血虚或瘀血阻碍，血不养心，心神不安，可致心悸怔忡。

《冯氏锦囊秘录•方脉惊悸怔忡健忘合参》说："怔忡者，心中跳动不安，惕惕如人将捕，有思虑便动者，皆属于血虚也。"指出心血不足，血不养心，是引起心动不安，心悸怔忡的病机。

《辨证录•惊悸门》说："夫魂魄不定而惊生，魂魄不安而悸起，皆心肝二部之血虚也。血虚则神无所归，魂无所主。"指出心血虚，血不养神，魂魄不定，则生惊悸。

《景岳全书•杂证谟•不寐》说："无邪而不寐者，必营气不足也。营主血，血虚则无以养心，心虚则神不守舍，故或为惊惕，或为恐畏，或若有所系恋，或无因而偏多妄思，以至终夜不寐，及忽寐忽醒，为鬼神不安等证。"指出心血不足，血不养神，神不守舍，魂魄外游，可致失眠多梦。

《杂病源流犀烛•心病源流》说："心为身之主，统领血海，故心血少则神不定，寝不安，百病集作。"指出心主血脉，心血虚弱，血不养神，神魂不定，可致失眠。

《古今医统》说："心为栖神之所，凡思虑过多，则心血亏耗而神游于外，故多梦。"精辟地论述了心血不足，神游于外，引起失眠多梦的病机。

《证治汇补•惊悸怔忡》说："有胸中痞塞，不欲饮食，心中常有所欠，爱居暗室，或倚门见人，即惊避无地，似失志状，此为卑谍之病。由心血不足者，人参养荣汤。"指出心血不足，不能养神，精神错乱，可引起焦虑恐惧、心悸不安等症。

10.4   Blood Vacuity with Visceral Agitation

When heart blood is insufficient, the liquids are depleted and the blood is scant. Blood vacuity causes visceral agitation because the body of the heart does not receive nourishment. The spirit qì loses its ability to govern itself and is unable to restrain the activities of the spirit-affect. This can lead to abstraction and instability of the essence-spirit. It manifests as frequent, uncontrollable sorrow with a desire to weep. In severe cases, abnormal speech will result.

At the same time, blood vacuity visceral agitation causes vacuity heat to stir and harass the heart spirit. This causes a disquieted heart spirit, which gives rise to vexation in the heart, derangement, unquiet sleep, and forgetfulness. These pathological changes of the spirit-mind are for the most part due to heart qì insufficiency, damage to the heart and spleen, failure of the blood to nourish the heart, and loss of enrichment to the visceral yīn.

Zhāng Zhòng-Jǐng referred to this condition as "visceral agitation disease." It should be treated by nourishing heart blood and quieting the heart spirit. For a formula, use Licorice, Wheat, and Jujube Decoction (*gān mài dà zǎo tāng*) from the *Jīn Guì Yào Lüè* ("Essential Prescriptions of the Golden Coffer"), with the addition of spiny jujube and polygala. This formula employs licorice and wheat to fortify the spleen and boost qì, and jujube to supplement the spleen and boost blood. By regulating the center and boosting qì, it supplements heart blood to quiet the spirit and stabilize the mind.

Licorice, Wheat, and Jujube Decoction (甘麦大枣汤 *gān mài dà zǎo tāng*)
gān cǎo (甘草 Glycyrrhizae Radix, licorice) *xiǎo mài* (浮小麦 Tritici Fructus, wheat) *dà zǎo* (大枣 Jujubae Fructus, jujube) Plus: *suān zǎo rén* (酸枣仁 Ziziphi Spinosi Semen, spiny jujube) *yuǎn zhì* (远志 Polygalae Radix, polygala)

血虚脏躁

心血不足，津亏血少，血虚脏躁，心体不得滋养，神气失去自主功能，不能控制神情活动，可引起精神恍惚不定，表现为时常悲伤欲哭，不能自主，甚则言语失常；同时，由于血虚脏躁，虚热扰动，而致心神不安，可引起心中烦乱，夜卧不安，遇事健忘等症。此类神志病变，大多数是由于心气不足，心脾受损，血不养心，脏阴失滋所致，张仲景称为脏躁病。治宜养心血，安心神。方用《金匮要略》甘麦大枣汤（甘草、小麦、大枣）加酸枣仁、远志。此方以甘草、小麦健脾益气，大枣补脾益血，通过调中益气，而达到补益心血，安神定志的作用。

Literature Review of Blood Vacuity with Visceral Agitation

📖 *Jīn Guì Yào Lüè* ("Essential Prescriptions of the Golden Coffer"), "Chapter on the Pulses and Patterns of Women's Miscellaneous Diseases"

"Women with visceral agitation [have] joy, sorrow, and a desire to weep; they appear as if affected by spirits, with frequent yawning and stretching. Licorice, Wheat, and Jujube Decoction governs [this condition]."

The expression "visceral agitation" in this quotation is the object of much debate and disagreement. Wèi Niàn-Tíng points out, "women with visceral agitation must have suffered damage from joy or sorrow. They are unresponsive, weep abnormally in deep sorrow, and appear as if affected by spirits, but are unaware that this is not a condition of spirits. In fact, it is a pattern caused by blood vacuity and liquid collapse, causing emptiness in the viscera and agitation."

This indicates that these changes in the spirit-mind are manifestations of heart blood deprived of nourishment, with blood vacuity and visceral agitation.

文献评述

《金匮要略·妇人杂病脉证篇》说："妇人脏躁，喜、悲伤欲哭，象如神灵所作，数欠伸，甘麦大枣汤主之。"其中"脏躁"二字，看法不一，争论较大。魏念庭指出："妇人脏躁者，必喜悲伤,无所感融，悲哭无常，象如神灵所作，不知非神灵也，乃血虚而津亡，脏空而发躁之证也。"明确提出此种神志变化不定的表现为心血失养，血虚脏躁。

Summary of Heart Spirit Irregularities

1. Spirit Qì Insufficiency

   Devitalized essence-spirit, lack of concentration, delayed and dull responses, forgetfulness

2. Spirit Failing to Keep to its Abode

   Agitation and stirring of the heart spirit: Heart palpitations and fearful throbbing, fright, fear, and disquietude

   Spirit wandering outward: Insomnia and profuse dreaming

3. Blood Vacuity with Visceral Agitation

Loss of control over the essence-spirit: Abstraction of the spirit-mind, frequent and uncontrollable sorrow with desire to weep, abnormal speech

Disquieted heart spirit: Vexation in the heart and derangement, unquiet sleep, and forgetfulness

心神失调

神气不足 —— 精神不振，思想不集中，反应迟钝，健忘遗事。

神不守舍

心神躁动 —— 心悸怔忡，惊恐不安。

神游于外 —— 失眠多梦。

血虚脏躁

精神失控 —— 神志恍惚，时常悲伤欲哭，不能自主，言语失常。

心神不安 —— 心中烦乱，夜卧不安，遇事健忘。

10.5   Blood Vessels Deprived of Nourishment

The *Sù Wèn* ("Plain Questions"), in the "Treatise on the Engenderment of the Five Viscera," states, "The heart is connected with the vessels and its luxuriance is reflected in the complexion." The channels and vessels are the pathways for the movement of blood. Heart qì propels the blood to fill and nourish the channels and vessels. Blood moves through the entire body and supplies moisture to the offices, orifices, skin, and four limbs (the "offices" here refers to the nose, eyes, lips, tongue, and ears).

The exuberance or debility of heart blood influences the function of the tissues, organs, viscera, and bowels. It is reflected externally in the luster and sheen of the complexion. When heart blood is insufficient, it is unable to ascend to provide luxuriance to the head and eyes. The head is the location of clear yáng and the eyes rely on blood for vision. When the head and eyes are deprived of the nourishment and moisture of blood, there is dizziness and flowery vision.

If heart blood is insufficient and blood is unable to ascend to provide luxuriance to the face, the blood network vessels in the face lack fullness; this manifests as a pale white or withered yellow facial complexion. In cases of severe blood loss, the blood network vessels in the face become empty and the facial complexion becomes pale white without luster or suddenly changes to somber white.

When the mouth, lips and tongue are deprived of nourishment by heart blood and the blood network vessels lose fullness, the lips and tongue will be pale and the tongue body will be thin and shrunken. When heart blood is unable to move to supply the four limbs and nails, the limbs will be numb and the nails will lack luster.

If heart blood vacuity causes blood to fail to fill and nourish the vessels and channels, the blood vessels become empty and the bodies of the vessels shrink. This results in a fine and weak pulse. Suitable treatment focuses on supplementing heart blood. For a formula, use Four Agents Decoction (*sì wù tāng*) from the *Tài Píng Huì Mín Hé Jì Jú Fāng* ("Tài-Píng Imperial Grace Pharmacy Formulas"), with the addition of astragalus and ginseng.

Four Agents Decoction (四物汤 *sì wù tāng*)
dāng guī (当归 Angelicae Sinensis Radix, Chinese angelica)
chuān xiōng (川芎 Chuanxiong Rhizoma, chuanxiong)
bái sháo (白芍 Paeoniae Radix Alba, white peony)
shú dì huáng (熟地黄 Rehmanniae Radix Praeparata, cooked rehmannia)
Plus:
huáng qí (黄芪 Astragali Radix, astragalus)
rén shēn (人参 Ginseng Radix, ginseng)

Moreover, if heart blood is insufficient and fails to nourish the flesh and skin, the blood vacuity may cause skin dryness and the formation of wind. This leads to dry, rough, itchy, or scaling skin. This condition should be treated by supplementing blood and moistening dryness while dispelling wind and relieving itching. For a formula, use Chinese Angelica Drink (*dāng guī yǐn zǐ*) from the text *Dān Xī Xīn Fǎ* ("Dān-Xī's Heart-Approach").

Chinese Angelica Drink (当归饮子 *dāng guī yǐn zǐ*)
dāng guī (当归 Angelicae Sinensis Radix, Chinese angelica)
chuān xiōng (川芎 Chuanxiong Rhizoma, chuanxiong)
shēng dì huáng (生地黄 Rehmanniae Radix Exsiccata seu Recens, dried/fresh rehmannia)
bái sháo (白芍 Paeoniae Radix Alba, white peony)
fáng fēng (防风 Saposhnikoviae Radix, saposhnikovia)
jí lí (蒺藜 Tribuli Fructus, tribulus)
hé shǒu wū (何首乌 Polygoni Multiflori Radix, flowery knotweed)
huáng qí (黄芪 Astragali Radix, astragalus)
gān cǎo (甘草 Glycyrrhizae Radix, licorice)

血脉失养

《素问•五脏生成篇》曰："心之合脉也，其荣色也。"经脉是血液运行的通路，心气推动血液，充养经脉，运行全身，营润官窍、皮肤、四肢。心血盛衰，可影响脏腑组织器官的功能活动，同时以颜色光泽反映于外。心血不足，不能上荣于头目，头为清阳之位，目得血而能视，头目失于血的滋养濡润，则为头晕眼花。若心血不足，血不上荣于面，面部血络充盈不足，可见面色淡白或萎黄；大失血时，面部血络空虚，则为面色淡白无华，或突然面色苍白。口唇、舌质失却心血供养，血络失充，则为唇舌色淡、舌体瘦薄。心血不能营运四肢爪甲，则为肢体麻木、爪甲不荣。心血虚，血不充养经脉，血脉空虚，脉体变小，故脉来细弱。治宜补养心血。方用《太平惠民和剂局方》<u>四物汤</u>加黄芪、人参。

此外，心血不足，不养于肌肤，血虚肤燥，血虚生风，可引起皮肤干燥，或粗糙，皮肤瘙痒，脱屑等症。治宜养血润燥，祛风止痒。方用《丹溪心法》<u>当归饮子</u>（当归、川芎、生地、白芍、防风、白蒺藜、首乌、黄芪、甘草）。

Literature Review of Blood Vessels Deprived of Nourishment

📖 *Zá Bìng Yuán Liú Xī Zhú* ("Incisive Light on the Source of Miscellaneous Disease"), "The Source of Heart Disease"

"The heart governs blood and blood is essence. Heart qì is originally in a natural state of surplus and it is only when essence is damaged and blood is lost that the heart suffers from insufficiency. Thus, when blood is exuberant, the spirit-light is profound and unified; when blood is debilitated, the mind and qì are clouded."

This quotation points out that in insufficiency of heart blood, blood fails to ascend to nourish the head; this leads to dizziness.

📖 *Zhōng Yī Lín Zhèng Bèi Yào* ("Clinical Essentials of Chinese Medicine"), "Bright White Facial Complexion"

"When the face is white like paper, it means that heart qì is verging on expiry."

Heart qì verging on expiry refers to a condition of severe damage to heart qì. It most often occurs when severe sweating, severe vomiting, severe precipitation, severe blood loss, or severe damage to yīn-blood causes qì to follow the blood and desert. Because qì and blood are unable to ascend to provide nourishment, the condition presents with a white and lusterless face.

📖 *Yī Shù* ("Account of Medicine")

> "The heart governs the vessels. When the color of the nails is lusterless, it indicates heart debility."

This quotation points out that when the heart is debilitated and therefore unable to govern the blood in the vessels, the blood will fail to provide luxuriance to the nails. This results in pale white nails.

📖 *Bǐ Huā Yī Jìng* ("*Bǐ Huā* Medical Mirror"), "Section on the Heart"

> "In heart vacuity, insufficiency of blood invariably results in a weak left inch pulse."

The left inch pulse indicates the condition of the heart. When heart blood is insufficient, the vessels lose fullness and nourishment. Thus, the left inch pulse becomes fine and weak.

文献评述

《杂病源流犀烛•心病源流》说："心主血，血即精也。心气原自有余，特精伤而失血，心便不足。故血盛则神明湛一，血衰则志气昏蒙。"指出心血不足，不能上养于头，可致头晕。

《中医临证备要•面色㿠白》说："面白如纸，则为心气垂绝。"心气垂绝是心气大伤，多由大汗、大吐、大下、大失血、阴血大伤，气随血脱所致，气血不能上养，因而导致面白无华。

《医述》引《医参》云："心主脉，爪甲色不华则心衰矣。"指出心衰时心不主血脉，血不荣爪甲，可致爪甲淡白。

《笔花医镜•心部》说："心之虚，血不足也，脉左寸必弱。"左寸脉候心，心血不足，脉失充养，故左寸脉细弱。

Summary of Blood Vessels Deprived of Nourishment
1. Head and Eyes Deprived of Nourishment Dizziness and flowery vision
2. Face Deprived of Nourishment *Blood vacuity:* Pale white or withered-yellow facial complexion *Severe blood loss:* Pale white lusterless facial complexion *Yang collapse* Sudden somber white facial complexion
3. Mouth and Lips Deprived of Nourishment Pale white lips and tongue, thin shrunken tongue

4. Four Limbs Deprived of Nourishment

   Numbness in the limbs, lusterless nails

5. Loss of Fullness in the Blood Vessels

   Fine and weak pulse

6. Skin Deprived of Nourishment

   Dry or rough skin, itching and scaling of the skin

血脉失养

头目失养 —— 头晕眼花。

面失养

　　面色淡白、萎黄（血虚）。

　　面色淡白无华 （大失血）。

　　面色突然苍白 （亡阳）。

口唇失养 —— 唇舌色淡，舌体瘦薄。

四肢失养 —— 肢体麻木，爪甲不荣。

血脉失充 —— 脉来细弱。

皮肤失养 —— 皮肤干燥，或粗糙，皮肤瘙痒，脱屑。

10.6　Blood Vacuity with Floating Yáng

Since blood is the mother of qì, it is the vehicle for qì, as well as its internal guard. Severe damage to heart blood results from external wounds or flooding and spotting, profuse menstrual periods, or postpartum blood loss in women. It may also result after large sores rupture. When blood is vacuous, qì has nothing to rely on; thus, yáng qì cannot be guarded internally. This results in the pathomechanism of blood vacuity with floating yáng, which manifests as false heat.

When blood is vacuous and loses its constraining ability, yáng floats into the fleshy exterior. Qì in superabundance causes heat, which can result in hot skin and a red face or high fever.

The heart governs blood and constitutes the material foundation for the activity of the essence-spirit. When heart blood is insufficient, the heart spirit is deprived of nourishment, and heart vexation results. When blood is vacuous and yáng qì floats outward, construction yīn is not secured and the fluids are not guarded internally. This causes the patient to be bathed in sweat. When the sweating is extremely profuse, patients drink water to rescue themselves; thus, there will be thirst and thoughts of drinking.

When yáng qì floats outward because of blood vacuity, the pulse will have a floating, large, and scallion-stalk quality. This condition is markedly different from scorching heat in the qì aspect, as seen in exuberant heat of the yáng brightness channel qì. This latter condition manifests with great heat effusion, great sweating, great thirst, and a surging and large pulse.

Blood vacuity with floating yáng should be treated by supplementing qì and nourishing blood while constraining floating yáng. For a formula, choose Chinese Angelica Blood-Supplementing Decoction (*dāng guī bǔ xuè tāng*) from the *Nèi Wài Shāng Biàn Huò Lùn* ("Clarification of Perplexities About Internal and External Damage").

Chinese Angelica Blood-Supplementing Decoction
(当归补血汤 *dāng guī bǔ xuè tāng*)

huáng qí (黄芪 Astragali Radix, astragalus)
dāng guī (当归 Angelicae Sinensis Radix, Chinese angelica)

血虚阳浮

血为气之母，血是气的载体，又是气的内守。如果外受创伤，妇女崩漏，月经量多，产后失血，或大疮溃后，心血大伤，血虚气无所附，阳气不能内守，则可引起血虚阳浮的病机，出现一派假热的表现。

血虚失敛，阳浮肌表，气有余则是热，可致肌热面赤，或身发高热；心主血，为精神活动的物质基础，心血不足，心神失养，则心烦不安；血虚阳气外浮，不能固护营阴，津液不能内守，则汗出如洗；汗出太多，病人引水自救，则口渴思饮；血虚阳气外浮，则脉象浮大而芤。此与阳明经气热盛，出现大热、大汗、大渴、脉洪大等气分热炽的病机迥然有别，治宜补气养血，收敛浮阳。方选《内外伤辨惑论》当归补血汤（黄芪、当归）。

Literature Review of Blood Vacuity with Floating Yáng

📖 *Yī Fāng Kǎo* ("Medical Remedies Researched")

"When blood is replete, the body is cool. When blood is vacuous, the body is hot. This may be caused by encumbrance in the flesh from taxation or from physical labor. Vacuity of yīn-blood results in yáng alone controlling the body; this generates all the patterns. This pattern superficially resembles White Tiger [Decoction], but can be distinguished by the fact that the pulse is large and vacuous as opposed to large and long."

This quotation points out that the pathomechanism of blood vacuity with generalized heat effusion is rooted in yīn-blood vacuity with yáng qì floating outward. Since construction and blood are governed by the heart, the pathomechanism of heart vacuity with floating yáng appears when heart blood is insufficient.

文献评述

《医方考》说："血实则身凉，血虚则身热。或以肌困劳役，虚其阴血，则阳独治，故诸证生焉。此证纯象白虎，但脉大而虚，非大而长为辨耳。"指出血虚身热的病机是阴血虚而阳气外浮，营血为心所主，所以心血不足时，可见血虚阳浮的病机。

Summary of Blood Vacuity with Floating Yáng
1. Yang Floating into the Fleshy Exterior   Heat effusion with a red face
2. Outward Discharging of Construction-Yīn   Sweating as if being bathed in sweat
3. Failure of the Heart to Nourish the Spirit   Heart vexation
4. Sweat Damaging Liquids   Vexing thirst with fluid intake
5. Loss of Constraint in the Vessel Qì   Floating, large, scallion-stalk pulse
血虚阳浮
阳浮肌表 —— 发热面赤。
营阴外泄 —— 汗出如洗。
心不养神 —— 心烦不安。
汗出伤津 —— 烦渴引饮。
脉气失敛 —— 脉浮大而芤。

When the pathomechanism of heart blood vacuity progresses to a more advanced state, it can result in pathological changes such as heart-liver blood vacuity, dual vacuity of heart qì and heart blood, or dual vacuity of yīn and blood.

Heart–Liver Blood Vacuity

The heart governs blood; the liver stores blood. When heart blood is vacuous and unable to provide blood to the liver for storage, the disease of the heart affects the liver. This can result in an insufficiency of liver blood, and in a more advanced state, can form the pathomechanism of heart-liver blood vacuity. The patient will present with a pale face, pale lips and tongue, heart palpitations and insomnia, as well as impaired vision, numbness in the limbs, and lusterless nails.

Dual Vacuity of Heart Qì and Heart Blood

The blood transforms qì. When heart blood is vacuous, blood fails to transform qì; this can result in heart qì vacuity. Conversely, when heart qì is insufficient, qì fails to engender blood, resulting in heart blood vacuity. The pathomechanism of dual vacuity of heart qì and heart blood arises from either process.

A patient with this condition will present with heart palpitations and shortness of breath, fatigued spirit and lack of strength, as well as insomnia, profuse dreaming, a pale face, and pale lips and tongue.

Dual Vacuity of Heart Yīn and Heart Blood

Blood is associated with yīn. When heart blood is vacuous, the construction-yīn inside the blood is reduced. This can result in heart yīn vacuity that advances to lead to a pathomechanism of dual vacuity of heart yīn and heart blood. Patients will present with heart palpitations, insomnia, and pale face, lips, and tongue, in conjunction with vexing heat in the five hearts or tidal heat and night sweating.

The blood belongs to yīn. Thus, when heart blood is vacuous, the construction-yin in the blood becomes diminished and heart yīn vacuity results. This causes the pathomechanism of dual vacuity of heart yīn and blood to arise. Patients manifest with heart palpitations, insomnia, pale lips and a pale face, as well as vexing heat in the five hearts, tidal heat, and night sweating.

心血虚的病机进一步发展，可引起心肝血虚，心的气血两虚、阴血两虚等病机变化。

心肝血虚：心主血，肝藏血。心血虚，不能提供血液为肝所藏，心病及肝，可引起肝血不足，进而发展形成心肝血虚的病机。病人既有面唇舌淡、心悸失眠，又有视减肢麻、爪甲不荣等表现。

心的气血两虚：血能化气，心血虚，血不化气，可引起心气虚；心气不足，气不生血，亦可引起心血虚，从而形成心的气血两虚病机。病人心悸气短、神疲乏力，与失眠多梦、面唇舌淡等症同见。

心的阴血两虚：血属阴，心血虚，血中营阴减少，可以导致心阴虚，进而引起心的阴血两虚病机。病人既有心悸失眠，面唇舌淡，同时伴见五心烦热，潮热盗汗等症。

Chapter Eleven

Heart Yīn Vacuity

The pathomechanisms of heart yīn vacuity began to be explored in a general way during the period of the *Huáng Dì Nèi Jīng* ("The Yellow Emperor's Inner Canon"). The *Shāng Hán Zá Bìng Lùn* ("On Cold Damage and Miscellaneous Diseases") contains related discussions in the section on heart vexation and insomnia in lesser yīn heat transformation patterns, as well as in the treatment of heart stirring and palpitations associated with Honey-Fried Licorice Decoction (*zhì gān cǎo tāng*). These discussions involve the pathomechanism of heart yīn vacuity indirectly.

The text *Wài Tái Mì Yào* ("Essential Secrets from Outside the Metropolis"), in the chapters on "Vacuity Taxation" and "Formulas for Heart Taxation Repletion Heat," contains a discussion of heart taxation as one of the five taxations: "Heart taxation [manifests as] incessant heat, scorched flesh and body hair, a complexion without moisture, a red and dry mouth, and oppression in the heart." By recommending "Ophiopogon Beverage" as a treatment, it constitutes a profound exposition of the pathomechanism of heart yīn vacuity.

During the Sòng, Jīn, and Yuán periods, the theory of yīn vacuity was developed extensively. Zhū Dān-Xī, the great master of the School of Nourishing Yīn, created the famous expression "yīn is constantly insufficient." He compounded famous formulas for enriching yīn and downbearing fire, such as Major Yīn Supplementation Pill (*dà bǔ yīn wán*) and Fine Jade Paste (*qióng yù gāo*), but he focused primarily on the study of liver-kidney yīn vacuity.

In the Míng period, Zhāng Jǐng-Yuè pointed out in a discussion on the pathomechanisms of fearful throbbing that "this symptom is only found in people with yīn vacuity taxation detriment." This is mentioned in the text *Jǐng Yuè Quán Shū* ("Jǐng-Yuè's Complete Compendium"), in the section "Schema of Miscellaneous Patterns: Fearful Throbbing, Fright, and Fear." When considering this statement in connection with the disease location of fearful throbbing, this can be considered as an indirect discussion of the pathomechanism of heart yīn vacuity.

Qín Jǐng-Míng's text *Zhèng Yīn Mài Zhì* ("Pathoconditions: Causes, Pulses, and Treatments"), in the section on "Insomnia due to Heart Blood Vacuity," includes a paragraph that describes the pathomechanism of heart blood vacuity: "The symptoms of insomnia due to heart blood vacuity are heart vexation, agitation, and derangement, awakening at night with fright, dryness of the mouth and tongue, and vexation heat in the five hearts." Considered as a whole, the manifestations in this paragraph do not refer to heart blood vacuity, but are symptoms representative of heart yīn vacuity. When mentioning the treatment methods, he again states: "In the treatment of insomnia due to heart blood vacuity, yīn is vacuous and yáng is therefore effulgent; this causes an insufficiency of heart blood. This is a pathocondition of fire. One should invigorate the governor of water to restrain the brilliance of yáng. The suitable treatment is to enrich yīn and downbear fire." This can be considered as the most in-depth and comprehensive early description of the pathomechanism of heart yīn vacuity. It is unfortunate that Mr. Qín mistook blood for yīn and turned heart yīn vacuity into heart blood vacuity, thus never directly mentioning the term heart yīn vacuity.

Lǐ Yòng-Cuì's *Zhèng Zhì Huì Bǔ* ("A Supplement to Patterns and Treatment"), from the Qīng dynasty, contains similar statements in a discussion on fright palpitations and fearful throbbing. It explains rather indiscriminately: "When yīn qì is internally vacuous, effulgent vacuity fire stirs."

It is only in modern times that the term heart yīn vacuity has been put forward clearly. For example, in the text *Pú Fǔ Zhōu Yī Liáo Jīng Yàn* ("Pú Fǔ-Zhōu's Medical Experience"), in the section on "Identifying Patterns and Seeking Roots," it states: "Heart yīn vacuity causes heart vexation, night sweating, a dry mouth and a red-tipped tongue, and possibly low-grade fever and forgetfulness." The pathomechanism and pattern of heart yīn vacuity have only now become generally accepted and widely employed, after being defined clearly in the national advanced college-level teaching materials.

The formation of heart yīn vacuity is usually caused by emotional dissatisfaction, fire transformation due to excess among the five minds, and qì and fire depressing internally; these factors invisibly wear on heart yīn. Alternatively, heart yīn vacuity may be caused by prolonged illness that excessively taxes the heart. This deprives the heart of nourishment and gradually wears on heart construction, damaging heart yīn. Heart yīn vacuity may also arise from warm-heat disease, if heat enters the construction aspect of the heart and scorches heart yīn.

Additional causes of heart yīn vacuity include: vomiting, diarrhea, sweating, blood loss, prolonged or severe illness, depletion of liquids in old age, or lack of treatment or inappropriate treatment. Pathological changes in the heart viscus itself can cause depletion damage as well. Such changes include damage from hyperactive heart fire, lack of nourishment because of insufficiency of heart blood, and devitalized heart qì and heart yáng that prevent transformation and engenderment.

Finally, changes transmitted from the other bowels and viscera can affect heart yīn. Examples include spleen-stomach vacuity causing insufficient engenderment and transformation, and liver-kidney yīn depletion preventing yīn from ascending to nourish the upper body.

The fundamental component in the pathomechanism of heart yīn vacuity is the loss of the heart's nourishing function. Because yīn and yáng are thrown off balance at the same time, internally engendered vacuity heat often results. In critical cases, there may be fulminant desertion of heart yīn.

心阴虚

《黄帝内经》时代已开始对阴虚病机作了广泛而粗略的概述。《伤寒杂病论》中少阴热化证的心烦不寐，以及用炙甘草汤治疗心动悸等有关论述，已逐步涉及到心阴虚的病机。《外台秘要•虚劳•心劳实热方》关于五劳中心劳的论述："心劳热不止，肉毛焦，色无润，口赤干燥，心闷，"并用<u>麦门冬饮</u>治疗，是对心阴虚病机的深入阐说。宋金元时期，阴虚学说有了较大发展，一代养阴派大师朱丹溪，虽有"阴常不足"等著名论述，创造了大补阴丸、琼玉膏等滋阴降火名方，但是主要侧重于探讨肝肾阴虚。直到明代张景岳在讨论怔忡病机时提出"此证惟阴虚劳损之人有之"（《景岳全书•杂证谟•怔忡惊恐》），结合怔忡的病位，可以认为是对心阴虚病机的间接论述。

秦景明《症因脉治•心血虚不得卧》对心血虚的病机有一段描述，他说："心血虚不得卧之症，心烦躁乱，夜卧惊起，口燥舌干，五心烦热。"从整体而论，此段表现并非心血虚所为，应是心阴虚的典型症状。特别在谈到治法时又说："心血虚不得卧之治，阴虚则阳必旺，故心血不足，皆是火症，宜壮水之主，以制阳光，治宜滋阴降火。"因此，可以认为，这是对心阴虚病机的最深刻、最全面的论述。可惜秦氏以血为阴，把心阴虚提成心血虚，未直接点出心阴虚的名称。清代李用粹《证治汇补》对惊悸怔忡讨论时亦有类似提法，但仍较为笼统地说成："阴气内虚，虚火旺动"（《证治汇补•惊悸怔忡》）。迄至近代才较为明确地提出心阴虚的名称，如《蒲辅周医疗经验•辨证求本》中说："心阴虚，则心烦，盗汗，口干，舌尖红，或见低热，健忘。"在全国高等院校统编教材中，对心阴虚的病机及证候作了准确的界定，才被大家公认和广泛应用。

　　心阴虚的形成，常由情志不遂，五志化火，气火内郁，暗耗心阴；或由久病失养，劳心过度，心营渐耗，损伤心阴；或于温热疾病，热入心营，灼伤心阴；或因呕吐下利，出汗失血，久病重病，年老津亏，失治误治，耗及心阴；心脏自身病变，如心火亢盛损伤，或心血不足，不能滋养，或心气、心阳不振，不能化生，均可引起心阴亏损；其它脏腑疾病的传变，如脾胃虚弱，生化不足，或肝肾阴亏，不能上养，亦可波及心阴，引起心的阴虚。心阴虚的基本病机是失于滋养；同时由于阴阳平衡失调，可引起虚热内生；严重时还可引起心阴暴脱。

11.1   Loss of Enrichment and Nourishment

Heart yīn refers to the yīn humor of the heart. Since blood is ascribed to yīn and contains fluids, heart yīn also includes construction-blood and is linked to blood in an inseparable relationship. The most central function of heart yīn is to nourish the heart spirit, the blood vessels, and the tissues, offices, and orifices [the "offices" here refers to the nose, eyes, lips, tongue, and ears, which overlap with the "orifices"]. When heart yīn is insufficient, it fails to nourish. This leads to pathological changes resulting in irregularities of the heart spirit, blood vessels deprived of nourishment, and loss of moisture in the body, offices, and orifices.

失于滋养

　　心阴是指心的阴液。由于血属阴，血中含有津液，故心阴亦包括营血在内，与血有着不可分割的联系。心阴主要对心神、血脉和全身组织官窍起着滋养作用。心阴不足，失于滋养，可引起心神失调，血脉失养和形体官窍失润的病机变化。

11.1.1   Irregularities of the Heart Spirit

The activities of the heart spirit are associated with yáng. By nature, heart yáng is easily stirred. Heart yáng relies on nourishment from heart yīn, which functions as the internal guard that envelops and contains the heart spirit. This is necessary to allow the spirit-mind to obtain peace and clear stillness.

　　When heart yīn is vacuous, the heart spirit loses its nourishment. Yīn fails to constrain yáng, so yáng qì floats and stirs, harassing the heart spirit. This results in a disquieted heart spirit, manifesting with heart palpitations, fearful throbbing, fright, and fear. If heart yīn is insufficient and yīn fails to contain yáng, yáng fails to enter yīn. Thus, the spirit fails to keep to its abode and the spirit and the ethereal soul wander outward, resulting in insomnia, profuse dreaming, and unquiet sleep.

If heart yīn is depleted, yīn fails to nourish the spirit; thus, thought is weakened and memory is poor. This results in forgetfulness and should be treated by nourishing heart yīn. For a formula, use Celestial Emperor Heart-Supplementing Elixir (*tiān wáng bǔ xīn dān*) from the *Shè Shēng Mì Pōu* ("Penetrating the Secrets of Life Cultivation").

Celestial Emperor Heart-Supplementing Elixir
(天王补心丹 *tiān wáng bǔ xīn dān*)

rén shēn (人参 Ginseng Radix, ginseng)

xuán shēn (玄参 Scrophulariae Radix, scrophularia)

dān shēn (丹参 Salviae Miltiorrhizae Radix, salvia)

shēng dì huáng (生地黄 Rehmanniae Radix Exsiccata seu Recens, dried/fresh rehmannia)

tiān dōng (天冬 Asparagi Radix, asparagus)

mài dōng (麦冬 Ophiopogonis Radix, ophiopogon)

bǎi zǐ rén (柏子仁 Platycladi Semen, arborvitae seed)

suān zǎo rén (酸枣仁 Ziziphi Spinosi Semen, spiny jujube)

yuǎn zhì (远志 Polygalae Radix, polygala)

wǔ wèi zǐ (五味子 Schisandrae Fructus, schisandra)

dāng guī (当归 Angelicae Sinensis Radix, Chinese angelica)

jié gěng (桔梗 Platycodonis Radix, platycodon)

zhū shā (朱砂 Cinnabaris, cinnabar)

fú líng (茯苓 Poria, poria)

心神失调

心神活动属阳，其性易动。必赖以心阴的滋养，作为内守，包涵心神，神志才得安宁、清静。心阴虚，心神失养，阴不制阳，阳气浮动，扰动心神，心神失宁，则为心悸怔忡、惊恐不安。若心阴不足，阴不涵阳，阳不入阴，神不守舍，神魂外游，则为失眠多梦，夜卧不宁。若心阴亏虚，阴不养神，神思减弱，记力减退，则可引起健忘。治宜滋养心阴。方用《摄生秘剖》天王补心丹（人参、玄参、丹参、生地、天冬、麦冬、柏子仁、酸枣仁、远志、五味子、当归、桔梗、朱砂、茯苓）。

Literature Review of Irregularities of the Heart Spirit

📖 *Jǐng Yuè Quán Shū* ("Jǐng-Yuè's Complete Compendium"), "Schema of Miscellaneous Patterns: Fearful Throbbing, Fright and Fear"

"The disease of fearful throbbing manifests with vibrations and stirring in the heart and chest, as well as apprehensive jerking and anxiety without a moment of quietude. This pattern exists only in people with damage from vacuity taxation. Yīn vacuity in the lower body causes qì to be unrooted and unable to return to its source. Thus, in the upper body, qì floats and vibrates in the chest and armpits; in the lower body, it quivers in the area around the umbilicus."

This quotation refers to yīn vacuity in the lower body, which invariably causes qì to ascend to damage heart yīn. This causes the heart spirit to be harassed, resulting in fright palpitations.

📖 *Zhèng Zhì Huì Bǔ* ("A Supplement to Patterns and Treatment"), "Fright Palpitations and Fearful Throbbing"

"Man is governed by the heart. …An internal vacuity of yīn qì gives rise to frenetic stirring of vacuity fire with heart palpitations and emaciation."

This quotation points out that vacuity detriment of heart yīn causes yīn to fail to restrain yáng. Thus, vacuity fire harasses and disquiets the heart spirit; this results in the subjective sensation of palpitations in the heart. Emaciation results when heart yīn is vacuous and unable to nourish the entire body.

📖 *Jǐng Yuè Quán Shū* ("Jǐng-Yuè's Complete Compendium"), "Schema of Miscellaneous Patterns: Sleeplessness"

"Sleep is rooted in yīn and governed by the spirit. When the spirit is quiet, there is sleep; when the spirit is disquiet, there is sleeplessness. Disquietude may be due to harassment by evil qì or an insufficiency of construction qì. …Sleeplessness in the absence of evil is due to insufficiency of construction-blood."

The construction-blood of the heart includes heart yīn. When heart yīn is insufficient, the spirit fails to be confined internally. This causes sleeplessness.

📖 *Zhèng Yīn Mài Zhì* ("Pathoconditions: Causes, Pulses, and Treatments"), "Heart Blood Vacuity and Inability to Sleep"

"Heart blood vacuity with inability to sleep is caused by curved movement of the spirit dynamic wearing out heart blood. When yáng fire is effulgent within yīn, the spirit-light is harassed internally and the heart spirit is disquiet. Hence, the symptom of sleeplessness arises."

From the phrases, "wearing out of heart blood" and "effulgent yáng fire within yīn," we can see that this condition is not caused purely by blood vacuity alone. Rather, this pathomechanism is due to a detriment of heart yīn that causes yīn to fail to restrain yáng. This, in turn, causes yáng to engender hyperactive fire, which harasses the spirit light.

📖 *Luó Shì Huì Yuē Yī Jìng* ("Luo's Brief Essence of Medical Mirror"), "On Fearful Throbbing, Fright Palpitations, and Forgetfulness"

> "Forgetfulness is caused by a noninteraction of the heart and kidney. Thus, in performing tasks, such patients fail to complete what they have begun, and in their speech, do not know the beginning or end [of a sentence]. This should be treated by supplementing the kidney and conducting it to interact above while nourishing the heart and causing it to downbear into the lower body. When water and fire interact and assist each other, forgetfulness will not occur."

This quotation points out that when kidney yīn is unable to ascend to nourish heart yīn, heart yīn becomes insufficient and is unable to nourish the spirit. Forgetfulness results when the spirit fails to govern the memory.

📖 *Biàn Zhèng Lù* ("Record of Pattern Identification"), "Entry on Forgetfulness"

> "When kidney water is provided to the heart, intelligence is engendered ceaselessly. When heart fire is provided to the kidney, the intelligence is engendered inexhaustibly. However, if heart fire is hyperactive, the kidney will fear the fire and will not dare to interact with the heart. If kidney water is exhausted, the heart will abhor the dryness of the water and will not dare to interact with the kidney When the two organs fail to interact with each other, they will invariably forget about each other."

When kidney yīn is depleted, kidney water is unable to ascend to nourish heart yīn. When heart fire is hyperactive, it is unable to descend and downbear. Thus, the heart and kidney stop interacting, causing forgetfulness. Although the root originates in the lower part of the body, the detriment affects heart yīn, depriving the heart spirit of nourishment. This is what leads to forgetfulness.

文献评述

《景岳全书•杂证谟•怔忡惊恐》说："怔忡之病，心胸筑筑振动，惶惶惕惕，无时得宁者是也。…此证惟阴虚劳损之人乃有之。盖阴虚于下，则守气无根，而气不归源，所以在上则浮撼于胸臆，在下则振动于脐旁。"此虽源于在下的阴虚，必上损心阴，方可扰动心神而作惊悸。

《证治汇补•惊悸怔忡》说："人之所主者心，…阴气内虚，虚火妄动，心悸体瘦 。"指出心阴虚损，阴不制阳，虚火扰动，心神不宁，而自觉心中悸动；心阴虚，不能滋养全身，可致形体消瘦。

《景岳全书•杂证谟•不寐》说："盖寐本乎阴，神其主也，神安则寐，神不安则不寐。其所以不安者，一由邪气扰，一由营气不足耳。…无邪而不寐，心之营血之不足也。"心之营血，包括心阴，心阴不足，神不内守，故致失眠。

《症因脉治•心血虚不得卧》说："心血虚不得卧之因，曲运神机，心血耗尽，阳火旺于阴中，则神明内扰，而心神不宁，不得卧之症作矣。"从"心血耗尽，阳火旺于阴中"可看出，已不是单纯血虚所为，已包含心阴的损耗，才能产生阴不制阳，阳亢生火，扰动神明的病机。

《罗氏会约医镜•论怔忡惊悸恐惧健忘》说："健忘者，心肾不交也。为事有始无终，言谈不知首尾。治宜补肾而使之上交，养心而使之下降，则水火交济，何健忘之有"指出肾阴不能上养心阴，心阴不足，不能养神，神不主记忆，而致健忘。

《辨证录•健忘门》说："肾水资于心，则智慧生生不息；心火资于肾，则智慧生生无穷；苟心火亢，则肾畏火而不敢交于心；肾水竭，则心恶水干而不肯交于肾，两不相交，则势必至于两相忘矣。"肾阴亏损，肾水不能上养心阴，心火亢不能下降，心肾失交，则作健忘。虽然本源在下，但必损及心阴，心神失养，才可能遇事善忘。

11.1.2 Heart Vessels Deprived of Nourishment

The heart governs the blood and vessels. The yīn humor in the blood has the function of moistening and nourishing the heart vessels. When heart yīn is worn and damaged, the fluids inside the blood are scant. Alternatively, if insufficiency of heart yīn causes yīn to be vacuous and generate heat, vacuity heat will blaze internally and wear on construction-yin. This causes the blood to congeal and become concentrated, sticky, and dense; the movement of blood becomes slow, obstructed, and rough to the point of stasis obstruction. This condition is referred to as "yīn vacuity with blood stasis."

If the body of the heart is deprived of nourishment and the blood does not circulate freely in the vessels, heart pain results. The text *Zá Bìng Yuán Liú Xī Zhú* ("Incisive Light on the Source of Miscellaneous Disease"), in the chapter on "The Origin of Heart Pain," states, "The heart governs all yáng, as well as yīn-blood. There is pain when there is evil and depression of yáng qì. Pain also results when yáng is vacuous and evil is exuberant. Evil and congealing of yīn-blood also cause pain. Pain also results from yīn vacuity with exuberant evil." This quotation is a relatively early reference to the pathomechanism of heart pain resulting from heart yīn vacuity.

In the section on "Chest Pain" in the contemporary text *Zhōng Yī Zhèng Hòu Zhěn Duǎn Zhì Liáo Xué* ("Chinese Medical Pattern Diagnosis and Treatment"), it is stated directly that the loss of nourishment by heart yīn can result in chest pain. When describing the pathomechanisms of chest pain, this text explains that "when heart yīn fails to nourish, it causes chest pain and chest oppression, heart palpitations and fearful throbbing, dryness in the mouth, vexation and agitation, sleeplessness and profuse dreaming, heat in the palms and soles, dizziness and tinnitus, a red-tipped tongue with scanty fur, and a fine and rapid pulse."

If heart yīn is depleted, it is unable to nourish. This deprives the heart vessels of nourishment and inhibits the movement of construction. Here, the pulse is fine or rough. Alternatively, if vacuity heat is engendered internally, vacuity fire drives the blood to move more quickly, resulting in a fine and rapid pulse. This should be treated by supplementing heart yīn while quickening blood and relieving pain. For a formula, choose Celestial Emperor Heart-Supplementing Elixir (*tiān wáng bǔ xīn dān*) from the *Shè Shēng Mì Pōu* ("Penetrating the Secrets of Life Cultivation"), with the addition of red peony, millettia, corydalis, and sandalwood.

Celestial Emperor Heart-Supplementing Elixir
(天王补心丹 *tiān wáng bǔ xīn dān*)

rén shēn (人参 Ginseng Radix, ginseng)

xuán shēn (玄参 Scrophulariae Radix, scrophularia)

dān shēn (丹参 Salviae Miltiorrhizae Radix, salvia)

shēng dì huáng (生地黄 Rehmanniae Radix Exsiccata seu Recens, dried/fresh rehmannia)

tiān dōng (天冬 Asparagi Radix, asparagus)

mài dōng (麦冬 Ophiopogonis Radix, ophiopogon)

bǎi zǐ rén (柏子仁 Platycladi Semen, arborvitae seed)

suān zǎo rén (酸枣仁 Ziziphi Spinosi Semen, spiny jujube)

yuǎn zhì (远志 Polygalae Radix, polygala)

wǔ wèi zǐ (五味子 Schisandrae Fructus, schisandra)

dāng guī (当归 Angelicae Sinensis Radix, Chinese angelica)

jié gěng (桔梗 Platycodonis Radix, platycodon)

zhū shā (朱砂 Cinnabaris, cinnabar)

fú líng (茯苓 Poria, poria)

Plus:

chì sháo (赤芍 Paeoniae Radix Rubra, red peony)

jī xuè téng (鸡血藤 Spatholobi Caulis, spatholobus)

yán hú suŏ (延胡索 Corydalis Rhizoma, corydalis)

tán xiāng (檀香 Santali Albi Lignum, sandalwood)

心脉失养

心主血脉，血中阴液有润养心脉的作用。心阴耗伤，血中津液减少，或心阴不足，阴虚生热，虚火内炽，营阴被耗，血液浓缩而粘稠，血行迟慢、滞涩渐致瘀阻，即所谓"阴虚血瘀"。如果心体失养，血脉不畅，则可引起心痛。如《杂病源流犀烛•心痛源流》说："夫心主诸阳，又主阴血，故因邪而阳气郁者痛，阳虚而邪盛者亦痛；因邪而阴血凝注者痛，阴虚而邪盛者亦痛。"较早提出心阴虚引起心痛的病机。

现代《中医证候诊断治疗学•胸痛》才直接指出心阴失养可引起胸痛。该书在论述胸痛的病机时说："心阴失养，胸痛胸闷，心悸怔忡，口干烦躁，失眠多梦，手足心热，头晕耳鸣，舌红少苔，脉细数。"若心阴亏损，不能滋养，血脉失充，营运不利，则脉来细涩；或有虚热内生，虚火逼迫，血液加快运行，则为脉细数。治宜补养心阴，活血止痛。方选《摄生秘剖》天王补心丹加赤芍、鸡血藤、玄胡、檀香。

Literature Review of Heart Vessels Deprived of Nourishment

📖 *Dú Yī Bǐ Jì* ("Notes in Reading Medical Books"), "Self-Biting and Manic Wandering [are Attributable to] Extreme Heat of Qì and Blood, Not Spirits"

> "The blood is like a boat and the fluids like the water. …The more the fluids are scorched and exhausted, the more the movement of blood becomes stagnant."

This quotation points out that an insufficiency of yīn-blood can result in blood stasis. The insufficiency causes the fluids in the blood to be scant; thus, the blood becomes sticky, thick, and slow-moving.

📖 *Yīn Xū Zhèng Zhì* ("Yīn Vacuity Patterns and Treatment"), "Heart Pain"

> "Heart pain ascribed to yīn vacuity is mostly located in the heart and kidney. …Unresolved sorrow and thought wear on heart yīn; yīn vacuity generates heat. Intense internal vacuity fire wears on construction-yīn, inhibits the heart vessels and creates heart pain."

This quotation describes in detail how the pathomechanism of heart pain due to yīn vacuity arises. Scantiness of liquid deprives the blood of enrichment, inhibiting its movement and obstructing the heart vessels.

📖 *Zhèng Yīn Mài Zhì* ("Pathoconditions: Causes, Pulses, and Treatments"), "Heart Blood Vacuity with Inability to Sleep"

"In cases of heart blood vacuity with inability to sleep, the pulse is fine and rapid in the left inch position and racing when the deep level is felt."

This statement actually points to heart yīn depletion causing the heart vessels to be deprived of nourishment, with concurrent harassment by vacuity fire. The left inch pulse governs the heart; here, its quality is fine and rapid.

文献评述

《读医笔记•自啮狂走是气血热极非祟也》说："夫血犹舟也，津液水也。""津液为灼竭，则血行愈滞。"指出阴血不足，血中津液减少，血液粘稠，运行迟慢，可致血瘀。

《阴虚证治•心痛》说："心痛属阴虚者，多在心肾。…忧思不解，暗耗心阴，阴虚生热，虚火内炽，营阴被耗，心脉不畅，发生心痛。"详细阐述阴虚引起心痛的病机是因津少失滋，血行不畅，心脉阻滞所致。

《症因脉治•心血虚不得卧》说："心血虚不得卧之脉，左寸细数，沉按多疾。"这里实际上是指心阴亏损，心脉失养，虚火扰动，主心的左寸脉出现细数之象。

11.1.3 Body, Offices, and Orifices Deprived of Nourishment

Heart yīn follows blood in its movement throughout the body. It nourishes and moistens the viscera and bowels, the five offices and nine orifices, and the four limbs and hundred bones. When heart yīn is depleted, it is unable to nourish the body, offices, and orifices ["offices" here refers to the five offices as used in a five-phase analogy: the nose, eyes, lips, tongue, and ears]. Externally, this presents with dryness in the mouth, nose, lips, and throat, a red tongue with scanty fur and lack of liquid, dry and rough skin, and brittle and lusterless hair. Internally, it manifests in short and scant urine, dry bound stool, and a fine pulse.

This condition should be treated by nourishing heart yīn to moisten the offices and orifices. For a formula, use Celestial Emperor Heart-Supplementing Elixir (*tiān wáng bǔ xīn dān*) from the *Shè Shēng Mì Pōu*

("Penetrating the Secrets of Life Cultivation"), with the addition of lily bulb, trichosanthes root, cooked rehmannia, and ass hide glue.

Celestial Emperor Heart-Supplementing Elixir (天王补心丹 *tiān wáng bǔ xīn dān*)
rén shēn (人参 Ginseng Radix, ginseng)
xuán shēn (玄参 Scrophulariae Radix, scrophularia)
dān shēn (丹参 Salviae Miltiorrhizae Radix, salvia)
shēng dì huáng (生地黄 Rehmanniae Radix Exsiccata seu Recens, dried/fresh rehmannia)
tiān dōng (天冬 Asparagi Radix, asparagus)
mài dōng (麦冬 Ophiopogonis Radix, ophiopogon)
bǎi zǐ rén (柏子仁 Platycladi Semen, arborvitae seed)
suān zǎo rén (酸枣仁 Ziziphi Spinosi Semen, spiny jujube)
yuǎn zhì (远志 Polygalae Radix, polygala)
wǔ wèi zǐ (五味子 Schisandrae Fructus, schisandra)
dāng guī (当归 Angelicae Sinensis Radix, Chinese angelica)
jié gěng (桔梗 Platycodonis Radix, platycodon)
zhū shā (朱砂 Cinnabaris, cinnabar)
fú líng (茯苓 Poria, poria)
Plus:
bǎi hé (百合 Lilii Bulbus, lily bulb)
tiān huā fěn (天花粉 Trichosanthis Radix, trichosanthes root)
shú dì huáng (熟地黄 Rehmanniae Radix Praeparata, cooked rehmannia)
ē jiāo (阿胶 Asini Corii Colla, ass hide glue)

形体官窍失养

心阴随血液运行全身脏腑组织，五官九窍，四肢百骸，发挥滋养、濡润作用。心阴亏损，不能滋养形体官窍，外见口鼻唇咽干燥、舌红少苔乏津、皮肤干涩、毛发枯槁的表现，内见小便短少、大便干结、脉细等症状。治宜滋养心阴，濡润官窍。方用《摄生秘剖》天王补心丹加百合、花粉、熟地、阿胶。

Summary of Loss of Enrichment and Nourishment
1. Loss of Nourishment in the Heart Spirit *Yang qì floating and stirring*: Heart palpitations, fearful throbbing, fright, and fear *Spirit failing to keep to its abode*: Sleeplessness and profuse dreaming, unquiet sleep

> *Weakening of the spirit-thought*: Reduced memory capacity or forget-fulness
>
> 2. Heart Vessels Deprived of Nourishment
>
> *Yin vacuity with blood stasis*: Heart and chest pain
> *Blood vessels deprived of nourishment*: A pulse that is fine and rough or fine and rapid
>
> 3. Formal Body Deprived of Nourishment
>
> *Loss of enrichment in the head and face*: Dry mouth, lips, nose, and throat, red tongue with scant liquid
> *Loss of enrichment in the skin and hair*: Dry rough skin, brittle and lusterless hair
> *Loss of enrichment affecting elimination*: Short and scant urine, dry bound stool

失于滋养
心神失养
阳气浮动 —— 心悸怔忡、惊恐。
神不守舍 —— 失眠多梦、夜卧不宁。
神思减弱 —— 记忆减退、健忘。
心脉失养
阴虚血瘀 —— 心胸疼痛。
血脉失养 —— 脉来细涩、细数。
形体失养
头面失滋 —— 口唇鼻咽干燥、舌红少津。
皮毛失滋 —— 皮肤干涩，毛发枯槁。
二便失滋 —— 小便短少，大便干结

11.2 Vacuity Heat Arising Internally

Heart yīn and heart yáng regulate and balance each other. When heart yīn has been damaged, it fails to help heart yáng. Thus, yáng becomes unrestrained and hyperactive. Because superabundant qì is fire, vacuity heat arises internally. When heart yīn is depleted, vacuity fire harasses the spirit, causing heart vexation. Since the heart is located in the chest, vacuity heat filling the chest causes a subjective sensation of heat and oppression in the chest.

The channels and vessels of the heart channel run along the throat and penetrate upward into the tongue. When heart yīn is vacuous and vacuity fire ascends to harass the lips and tongue, it can cause a dry sore throat, red dry lips, and a red-tipped tongue, as well as sores, bleeding, and ulceration of the mouth and tongue. If vacuity fire ascends to fill the blood vessels of the head and face, one can observe a red face and eyes.

Night is ascribed to yīn and sweat is the humor of the heart. In cases of heart yīn vacuity, the yīn vacuity and yáng hyperactivity are aggravated when night falls and defense yáng passes from the exterior into the interior. This causes outward floating of vacuous yáng and manifests in pathoconditions of tidal heat and night sweating. The hand lesser yīn channel runs to the palms of the hands and the foot lesser yīn channel penetrates to the soles of the feet. Thus, when heart yīn is depleted, one tends to see vexing heat in the five hearts.

This condition should be treated by supplementing heart yīn while clearing heat and draining fire. For a formula, use Celestial Emperor Heart-Supplementing Elixir (*tiān wáng bǔ xīn dān*) from the *Shè Shēng Mì Pōu* ("Penetrating the Secrets of Life Cultivation"), with the addition of coptis, anemarrhena, stellaria, lycium root bark, lily bulb, and oyster shell.

Celestial Emperor Heart-Supplementing Elixir
(天王补心丹 *tiān wáng bǔ xīn dān*)

rén shēn (人参 Ginseng Radix, ginseng)

xuán shēn (玄参 Scrophulariae Radix, scrophularia)

dān shēn (丹参 Salviae Miltiorrhizae Radix, salvia)

shēng dì huáng (生地黄 Rehmanniae Radix Exsiccata seu Recens, dried/fresh rehmannia)

tiān dōng (天冬 Asparagi Radix, asparagus)

mài dōng (麦冬 Ophiopogonis Radix, ophiopogon)

bǎi zǐ rén (柏子仁 Platycladi Semen, arborvitae seed)

suān zǎo rén (酸枣仁 Ziziphi Spinosi Semen, spiny jujube)

yuǎn zhì (远志 Polygalae Radix, polygala)

wǔ wèi zǐ (五味子 Schisandrae Fructus, schisandra)

dāng guī (当归 Angelicae Sinensis Radix, Chinese angelica)

jié gěng (桔梗 Platycodonis Radix, platycodon)

zhū shā (朱砂 Cinnabaris, cinnabar)

fú líng (茯苓 Poria, poria)

Plus:

huáng lián (黄连 Coptidis Rhizoma, coptis)

zhī mǔ (知母 Anemarrhenae Rhizoma, anemarrhena)

yín chái hú (银柴胡 Stellariae Radix, stellaria)

dì gǔ pí (地骨皮 Lycii Cortex, lycium bark)

bǎi hé (百合 Lilii Bulbus, lily bulb)

mǔ lì (牡蛎 Ostreae Concha, oyster shell)

虚热内生

心阴与心阳相互为用，协调平衡。心阴有损，不济心阳，阳失制约，心阳偏亢，气有余便是火，则致虚热内生。心阴亏损，虚火扰神，则为心烦不安。胸为心位，虚热充胸，自觉胸中热闷。

心经经脉循行咽候，上通于舌，心阴虚，虚火上扰唇舌，可为咽候干痛、唇红干燥、舌尖红、口舌生疮、出血、溃烂。虚火上升，头面血脉充盈，可见面红目赤。夜晚属阴，心在液为汗，心阴虚损，入夜之际，卫阳由表入里，加重阴虚阳亢的程度，虚阳外浮，故易见潮热盗汗之症。手少阴经脉行于掌心，足少阴经脉通足心，故心阴亏损者，易见五心烦热。治宜补养心阴，清热泻火。方用《摄生秘剖》天王补心丹加黄连、知母、银柴胡、地骨皮、百合、牡蛎。

Literature Review of Internal Generation of Vacuity Heat

📖 *Biàn Zhèng Lù* ("Record of Pattern Identification"), "Entry on Vacuity Vexation"

> "When kidney water interacts with the heart, there is peace. …The heart is quiet when [the heart and kidney] help each other; vexation results when they do not help each other. Old people tend to suffer from solitary yáng and lack of water, causing hot qì to surge upward. This actually refers to kidney fire surging up into the heart. Superabundance of fire actually means that water is insufficient."

This quotation explains that when kidney yáng is worn out, it is unable to ascend to nourish heart yīn. Heart fire stirs when heart yīn is vacuous, resulting in vacuity vexation.

📖 *Zhèng Zhì Huì Bǔ* ("A Supplement to Patterns and Treatment"), "Fright Palpitations and Fearful Throbbing"

> "Internal vacuity of yīn qì with frenetic stirring of vacuity fire is characterized by heart palpitations and emaciation, vexing heat in the five hearts, a red face and dry lips, and a left pulse that is faint and weak or vacuous, large, and forceless."

The effulgent yīn vacuity fire described in this text should be related to the pathomechanisms of heart yīn vacuity and vacuity fire harassing internally. This is based on the theory that the heart governs the blood vessels, its bloom is in the face, and the left inch pulse is ascribed to the heart; in addition, there is heart vexation and the channels in the palms connect with the heart in the upper body.

文献评述

《辨证录•虚烦门》说："肾水交心，而成既济之泰。…故既济而心安，未济而心烦耳。老人孤阳无水，热气上冲，乃肾火冲心。火之有余，实水之不足。"充分说明，肾阴耗损，不能上养心阴，心阴虚，心火扰动，可致虚烦。

《证治汇补•惊悸怔忡》云："有阴气内虚，虚火妄动，心悸体瘦，五心烦热，面赤唇燥，左脉微弱，或虚大无力者是也。"根据心主血脉，其华在面；左寸脉属心；心烦、手心的经脉上与心相关等理论，此文中所指阴虚火旺，应与心阴虚，虚火内扰的病机有关。

Summary of Vacuity Heat Arising Internally

1. Vacuity Heat Harassing the Spirit

   Heart vexation, oppression and heat in the heart
2. Ascending to Harass the Lips and Tongue

   Dry sore throat; red and dry lips; red-tipped tongue; sores, bleeding, and ulceration of the mouth and tongue
3. Ascending to Harass the Head and Face

   Red face and eyes
4. Generalized Vacuity Heat

   Vexing heat in the five hearts, tidal heat, and night sweating

虚热内生

虚热扰神 —— 心烦不安，心中闷热。
上扰唇舌 —— 咽候干痛、唇红干燥、舌尖红、口舌生疮、出血、溃烂
上扰头面 —— 面目红赤。
全身虚热 —— 五心烦热，潮热盗汗。

11.3 Fulminant Desertion of Heart Yīn

The text *Sù Wèn* ("Plain Questions"), in the "Treatise on the Arcane Book of the Orchid Chamber of the Spirit Tower," states, "The heart is the great governor of the five viscera and six bowels. …When the governor is bright, the subjects are safe. When the governor is not bright, the twelve offices are endangered."

Heart yīn is the material foundation for maintaining the activities of the heart spirit. High fever, severe sweating, severe vomiting, and severe blood loss can easily lead to a critical loss of heart yīn. When heart yīn is verging on desertion, it is unable to tie heart yáng, causing yīn exhaustion and yáng desertion. Thus, the spirit is without foundation, which easily gives rise to fulminant desertion of heart yīn and the dissipation and collapse of spirit-qì.

This process is involved in the critical pathomechanism of yīn collapse with spirit clouding. In addition to coma, one can observe profuse and incessant sweating, sweaty hot sticky hands, red lips and a crimson dry parched tongue, warm hands and feet, and a fine, rapid, and forceless pulse.

The text *Wēn Bìng Tiáo Biàn* ("Systematized Identification of Warm Diseases"), in the "Chapter on the Upper Burner," states, "In greater yīn warm disease, severe sweating is contraindicated. If sweating is excessive, it will cause clouding of the heart spirit and delirious speech." This refers to the pathomechanism of yīn collapse and stupor. Exuberant heat damages yīn, causing yīn exhaustion and desiccation of liquids. It should be treated by supplementing yīn and securing desertion. For a formula, use Pulse-Engendering Powder (*shēng mài sǎn*) from the *Nèi Wài Shāng Biàn Huò Lùn* ("Clarification of Perplexities about Internal and External Damage"), with the addition of dragon bone and oyster shell.

Pulse-Engendering Powder (生脉散 *shēng mài sǎn*)

rén shēn (人参 Ginseng Radix, ginseng)
mài dōng (麦冬 Ophiopogonis Radix, ophiopogon)
wǔ wèi zǐ (五味子 Schisandrae Fructus, schisandra)
Plus:
lóng gǔ (龙骨 Mastodi Ossis Fossilia, dragon bone)
mǔ lì (牡蛎 Ostreae Concha, oyster shell)

Fulminant desertion of heart yīn presents with coma, profuse and incessant sweating, sweaty hot sticky hands, red lips, a crimson dry parched tongue, warm hands and feet, and a fine, rapid, and forceless pulse.

When heart yīn vacuity advances even further, it can lead to such pathological changes as dual vacuity of heart yīn and heart yáng, dual vacuity of heart qì and heart yīn, or noninteraction of the heart and kidney.

Dual Vacuity of Heart Yīn and Heart Yáng

In heart yīn vacuity, when the detriment of yīn affects yáng, it can cause heart yáng vacuity. This forms dual vacuity of heart yīn and heart yáng (see the section on heart yáng vacuity).

Dual Vacuity of Heart Qì and Heart Yīn

In heart yīn vacuity, there is qì transformation failure or qì lacking support. The detriment affects heart qì, causing dual vacuity of heart qì and heart yīn (see heart qì vacuity).

Noninteraction of the Heart and Kidney

This occurs from heart yīn vacuity with upward flaming of heart fire. It may also result from heart yīn vacuity sapping kidney yīn, causing kidney yīn depletion. When water and fire fail to help each other, the result is noninteraction of the heart and kidney. In the upper body, this manifests with fright palpitations and insomnia. In the lower body, it manifests with aching lumbus and knees and seminal emission.

心阴暴脱

"心为五脏六腑之大主。…故 主明则下安，主不明则十二官危"（《素问•灵兰秘典》）。心阴是维系心神活动的物质基础，高热、大汗、大吐、大失血等诸多因素，最易导致心阴严重丢失。心阴欲脱，不系心阳，阴竭阳脱，神无依附，则易发生心阴暴脱，神气消亡，出现亡阴神昏的危重病机。除见神志昏迷外，还可见到大汗不止、汗热粘手、唇红舌绛干焦、手足温和、脉细数无力等表现。如《温病条辨•上焦篇》说："太阴温病，不可大汗…汗出过多，心神昏谵语。"此即热盛伤阴，阴竭津涸而引起的亡阴昏迷的病机。治宜补阴固脱。方用《内外伤辨惑论》生脉散加龙骨、牡蛎。

心阴暴脱神志昏迷，大汗不止、汗热粘手、唇红舌绛干焦、手足温和、脉细数无力。

心阴虚的病机进一步发展，可引起心的阴阳两虚，心的气阴两虚，心肾不交等病机变化。

心的阴阳两虚：心阴虚，阴损及阳，可致心阳虚，进而形成心的阴阳两虚（见心阳虚）。

心的气阴两虚：心阴虚，不能化气，或阴虚气无所附，损及心气，可引起心的气阴两虚（见心气虚）。

心肾不交：心阴虚，心火上炎，不能下降，或心阴虚，下汲肾阴，肾阴亏损，水火失济，易致心肾不交。上见惊悸失眠，下见腰膝酸痛、遗精等症。

Index

About the Authors

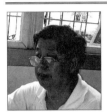

Yàn Shí Lín is a professor and Ph.D. advisor at Chengdu University of Traditional Chinese Medicine. He has enjoyed a distinguished professional career spanning more than 40 years with a specialization in pathomechanisms research and pattern differentiation. Among his Chinese published contributions he has written as Editor-in-Chief of the Diagnosis Chapter of the medical volume of the *Chinese Medical Encyclopedia,* the Pulse Diagnosis portion of the *Chinese Medical Classics* Series, and the *Study Guide Series for Self-Study Tests in Chinese Medicine.* He also contributed to the compilation of both the 6th and the 7th edition of the *Chinese National Standardized Textbooks* and the accompanying study guides, as well as many other national textbook projects. Additionally, he has published more than 80 academic papers in the field of Chinese medicine.

Academically, he has been the first to raise important theories such as cold-fire, sunken qì of liver and spleen, and qì stagnation caused by middle jiao vacuity. He has undertaken a thorough and detailed study of the pathomechanisms of the five zang as well as micro-modeling of zàng fǔ pattern differentiation in Chinese medicine that has contributed greatly to researching patterns in Chinese medicine.

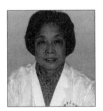

Lǐ Zhèng-Huà is Professor of Chinese Medicine and Dean of the Adult Education College at Chengdu University of Traditional Chinese Medicine. Professor Li also holds the Vice-Secretary position in the China National Chinese Medical Adult Education Association. She has accumulated more than 40 years of experience in teaching, scientific research, and clinical practice, with a specialization in internal medicine and pediatrics as well as many other types of complex clinical patterns, and is the author of three books and 27 academic papers in Chinese medicine.

Paradigm Publications

Recently Published Works

A Heart Approach to Gynecology: Essentials in Verse

The *Fù Kē Xīn Fǎ Yào Jué* is the gynecology section of the imperial compilation known as the *Golden Mirror of Orthodox Medicine*, a comprehensive, 90-volume compendium of medical theory and practice compiled by court physicians in 1742 and used as a text-book for the Imperial Medical School in the Qing Dynasty. The au-thors claimed that the *Golden Mirror* contained the core of Chinese medical doctrine; with this "bright, golden mirror," replete with vivid illustrations and effective therapies for many disorders, schol-ars might see clearly the origin and lineage of orthodox Chinese medicine.

Compared to other classics on gynecology, this work was both a relatively late arrival and relatively brief. Nonetheless, it rapidly gained favor among physicians. It is distinguished by its concise and well-expressed insights, which were presented in verses complemented by annotations. The text was highly regarded because it was a rigorous and scholarly work that covered a wide variety of gynecological issues in a manner that allowed the key clinical points to be rapidly assimilated. The formulas contained within were effective and were based upon generations of experience.

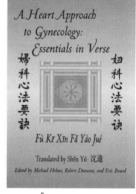

However, it is not just a medical classic of the past. Because it covers conditions that are timeless and common, and provides in-sights into the evolution of Chinese medical theory, it offers clini-cally useful tools for the modern day. It offers readers an under-standing of how to utilize many classical formulas and their varia-tions, and how to create their own formulas.

Paperback
336 pages
7"x10"
available
September 2005

It presents the most common topics related to women's health. Chapters are structured with verses followed by annotations and are dedicated to menstruation, fertility, pregnancy, childbirth, and postpartum care. Altogether, 161 classical formulas and their varia-tions are presented. Focusing on identifying yin and yang patterns of illness based on presenting signs, the *Fu Ke* investigates women's health in a clear and systematic way, epitomizing the sophisticated philosophy and style of Chinese medicine, drawing from major medical classics and presenting information in a concise way for easy learning.

Order from
Redwing Books
www.redwingbooks.com